HYGIENE AND SANITATION MANAGEMENT IN HOSPITALITY INDUSTRY

Karnail Singh

NAMAN PUBLISHER & DISTRIBUTORS
NEW DELHI

Published by
Sangeeta Jain for Naman Publisher & Distributors
7360-B, Prem Nagar,
Gali No.1, Shakti Nagar,
Delhi-110007
PH: 23823642, MOB.: 09013478302
E-mail: rajivjain72@ymail.com

Edition 2021

ISBN–978-81–920935–7-4

SOLE DISTRIBUTOR
JINDAL BOOK SERVICES
LG-4A, Ganpati Bhawan,
4675-B/21, Ansari Road,
Darya Ganj, Delhi - 110002

Jacket Designed by :
S.M. Graphics

Printed by:
Balaji Offset, Delhi 110032

Preface

In any food establishments, food handlers are either the first line of defense or the cause for the need for defense. This is because most types of foods can be contaminated and it is the responsibility of the food handler to ensure the safety of the consumers by eliminating or minimizing. In any food establishments, food handlers are either the first line of defense or the cause for the need for defense. This is because most types of foods can be contaminated and it is the responsibility of the food handler to ensure the safety of the consumers by eliminating or minimizing the contamination to safer levels for consumption. How to lessen, prevent, and eliminate contamination that causes food borne illness will be the focus of the study. Personal hygiene controls include all precautions taken by food handlers to protect food from contamination and to reduce the risk of food poisoning and food borne illness.

If good personal hygiene practices are not applied, food may be exposed to the risk of contamination. You need to have rules and procedures in place to ensure that your Personal Hygiene is effectively managed.

he contamination to safer levels for consumption. How to lessen, prevent, and eliminate contamination that causes food borne illness will be the focus of the study. Personal hygiene controls include all precautions taken by food handlers to protect food from contamination and to reduce the risk of food poisoning and food borne illness.

Sanitation management refers to the practices and procedures necessary to ensure a clean, safe establishment. Proper sanitation is important in any job, though it is especially valuable, and often enforced by law, in the food service, agriculture, and healthcare industries. Effective sanitation management requires skilled workers and supervisors to ensure that a facility maintains cleanliness and meets all regional and federal sanitation codes. Duties of sanitation workers may include physically cleaning facilities, training employees in sanitary practices, and conducting regular inspections.

Sanitation management in healthcare is similar to the practices found in the food service industry, though there is a special focus on sterilization and proper disposal of potentially harmful products. Healthcare workers are instructed to dispose of used needles, gauze, and other items in appropriate biohazard waste bins. Trained janitors may be asked to sterilize medical testing equipment and operating rooms in addition to performing standard cleaning jobs. In addition, regular health inspections by government officials are an important part of hospital sanitation management.

This book is designed and presented in an easy to read and easy to understand format. It will be beneficial to both aspiring professionals and those already in the industry.

We hope this text book meets its intended purpose as a practical resource, and serve as a vehicle for promoting the professionalism of this important segment of the Hospitality Industry.

KARNAIL SINGH

Contents

1

Cleaning and Sanitation

Water comprises approximately 95-99% of cleaning and sanitising solutions. The impurities in water can drastically alter the effectiveness of a detergent or a sanitiser. Water hardness is the most important chemical property with a direct effect on cleaning and sanitising efficiency. Water pH ranges generally from pH 5 to 8.5. This range is of no serious consequence to most detergents and sanitisers. However, highly alkaline or highly acidic water may require additional buffering agents. Water can also contain significant numbers of microorganisms.

Food soil is generally defined as unwanted matter on food-contact surfaces. Soil is visible or invisible. The primary source of soil is from the food product being handled. However, minerals from water residue and residues from cleaning compounds contribute to films left on surfaces. Microbiological biofilms also contribute to the soil buildup on surfaces. Since soils vary widely in composition, no one detergent is capable of removing all types. Many complex films contain: combinations of food components, surface oil or dust, insoluble cleaner components, and insoluble hard-water salts. These films vary in their solubility properties depending upon such factors as heat effect, age, dryness, time, etc. It is essential that personnel involved have an understanding of the nature of the soil to be removed before selecting a detergent or cleaning regime. Therule of thumb is that acid cleaners dissolve alkaline soils (minerals) and alkaline cleaners dissolve acid soils and food wastes.

Improper use of detergents can actually "set" soils, making them more difficult to remove (e.g., acid cleaners can precipitate protein). Many films and biofilms require more sophisticated cleaners which are amended with oxidising agents (such as chlorinated detergents) for removal. The physical condition of the soil deposits also effects its solubility. Freshly precipitated soil in a cool or cold solution is usually more easily dissolved than an old, dried, or baked-on deposit, or a complex film.

Fat: Fat usually is present as an emulsion and can generally be rinsed away with hot water above the melting point. More difficult fat and oil residues can be removed with alkaline detergents which have good emulsifying or saponifying ingredients.

Protein: In the food industry, proteins are by far the most difficult soils to remove. In fact, casein (a major milk protein) is used for its adhesive properties in many glues and paints. Food proteins range from more simple proteins, which are easy to remove, to more complex proteins, which are very difficult to remove. Heat-denatured proteins can be extremely difficult.

Carbohydrate: Simple sugars are readily soluble in warm water and are quite easily removed. Starch residues, individually, are also easily removed with mild detergents. Starches associated with proteins or fatscan usually be easily removed by highly alkaline detergents.

Mineral Salt: Mineral salts can be either relatively easy to remove, or be highly troublesome deposits or films. Calcium and magnesium are involved in some of the most difficult mineral films. Under conditions involving heat and alkaline pH, calcium and magnesium can combine with bicarbonates to form highly insoluble complexes.

Other difficult deposits contain iron or manganese. Salt films can also cause corrosion of some surfaces. Difficult salt films require an acid cleaner (especially organic acids which form complexes with these salts) for removal.

Microbiological films: Under certain conditions, microorgranisms (bacteria, yeasts, and molds) can form invisible films (biofilms) on surfaces. Biofilms can be difficult to remove and usually require cleaners as well as sanitisers with strong oxidising properties.

Lubricating greases and oils: These deposits (insoluble in water, alkali, or acid) can often be melted with hot water or steam, but oftenleave a residue. Surfactants can be used to emulsify the residue to make it suspendable in water and flushable.

Cleanability Surface

The cleanability of the surface is a primary consideration in evaluating cleaning effectiveness. Stainless steel is the preferred surface for food equipment and is specified in many industry and regulatory design and construction standards. Other "soft" metals (aluminum, brass, copper, or mild steel), or nonmetallic surfaces (plastics, or rubber) are also used on food contact surfaces. Surfaces of soft metals and nonmetallic materials are generally less corrosion- resistant and care should be exercised in their cleaning.

Aluminum is readily attacked by acids as well as highly alkaline cleaners which can render the surface non-cleanable. Plastics are subject to stress cracking and clouding from prolonged exposure to corrosive food materials or cleaning agents. Hard wood (maple or equivalent) or sealed wood surfaces should only be used in limited applications such as cutting boards or cutting tables provided the surface is maintained in good repair.

Such surfaces are more difficult to clean or sanitise, and may no longer be cleanable.

Detergents

Detergents and cleaning compounds are usually composed of mixtures of ingredients that interact with soils in several ways. In some detergents, specific enzymes are added to catalytically react with, and degrade, specific food soil components. The primary physically active ingredients are the surface active compounds termed surfactants. These organic molecules have general structural characteristicwhere a portion of the structure is hydrophilic (water- loving) and a portion is hydrophobic (not reactive with water). Such molecules function in detergents by promoting the physical cleaning actions through: emulsification, penetration, spreading, foaming, and wetting. It is a common practice to blend surfactant ingredients to optimise their properties. However, because of precipitation problems, cationic and anionic surfactants cannot be blended.

The most common inorganic acids used include: phosphoric, nitric, sulfamic, sodium acid sulfate, and hydrochloric. Organic acids, such as hydroxyacetic, citric, and gluconic, are also in use. Acid detergents are often used in a two-step sequential cleaning regime with alkaline detergents. Acid detergents are also used for the prevention or removal of stone films (mineral stone, beer stone, or milk stone).

Water conditioners are used to prevent the build-up of various mineral deposits (water hardness, etc.). These chemicals are usually sequestering agents or chelating agents. Sequestering agents form soluble complexes with calcium and magnesium. Examples are sodium tripolyphosphate, tetra-potassium pyrophosphate, organo-phosphates, and polyelectrolytes. Chelating agents include sodium gluconate and ethylene diamine tetracetic acid (EDTA).

Enzyme-based detergents, which are amended with enzymes such as amylases and other carbohydrate-degrading enzymes, proteases, and lipases, are finding acceptance in specialised food industry applications. The primary advantages of enzyme detergents are that they are more environmentally friendly and often require less energy input (less hot water in cleaning). Uses of most enzyme cleaners are usually limited to unheated surfaces (e.g., cold-milk surfaces). However, new generation enzyme cleaners (currently under evaluation) are expected to have broader application.

Fillers add bulk or mass, or dilute dangerous detergent formulations which are difficult to handle. Strong alkalis are often diluted with fillers for ease and safety of handling. Water is used in liquid formulations as a filler. Sodium chloride or sodium sulfate are often fillers in powdered detergent formuations.

Effective Sanitising

Effectiveness sanitising is dependant upon a number of factors including: initial contamination load, humidity, pH, temperature, and time. The use of steam as a sanitising process has limited application. It is generally expensive compared to alternatives, and it is difficult to regulate and monitor contact temperature and time. Further, the byproducts of steam condensation can complicate cleaning operations. Hot-water sanitising—through immersion (small parts, knives, etc.), spray (dishwashers), or circulating systems—is commonly used. The time required is determined by the temperature of the water.

The primary advantages of hot-water sanitisation are: relatively inexpensive, easy to apply and readily available, generally effective over a broad range of microorganisms, relatively non-corrosive, and penetratesinto cracks and crevices. Hot-water sanitisation is a slow process which requires come-up and cool-down time; can have high energy costs; and has certain safety concerns for employees. The process also has the disadvantages of forming or contributing to film formations, and shortening the life of certain equipment or parts thereof (gaskets, etc.).

The registration of chemical sanitisers and antimicrobial agents for use on food and food product contact surfaces, and on nonproduct contact surfaces, is through the U.S. Environmental Protection Agency (EPA). Thus, any antimicrobial agent and its maximum usage level for direct use on food or on food product contact surfaces must be approved by the FDA.

Prior to the sanitisation process, all surfaces must be clean and thoroughly rinsed to remove any detergent residue. An unclean surface cannot be sanitised. Since the effectiveness of sanitisation requires direct contact with the microorganisms, the surface should be free of cracks, pits, or crevices which can harbor microorganisms. Surfaces which contain biofilms cannot be effectively sanitised.

Generally, the activity of a sanitiser increases with increased concentration. However, a leveling off occurs at high concentrations. A common misconception regarding chemicals is that "if a little is good, more is better". Using sanitiser concentrations above recommendations does not sanitiser better and, in fact, can be corrosive to equipment and in the long run lead to less cleanability.

Sanitisers are dramatically affected by the pH of the solution. Many chlorine sanitisers, for example, are almost ineffective at pH values above 7.5. Organic and/or inorganic inactivators may react chemically with sanitisers giving rise to non-germicidal products. Some of these inactivators are present in detergent residue. Thus, it is important that surfaces be rinsed prior to sanitisation. The microbiological load can affect sanitiser activity. Also, the type of microorganism present is important. Spores are more resistant than vegetative cells. Certain sanitisers are more active against gram positive than gram negative microorganisms, and vice versa.

Chlorine, in its various forms, is the most commonly used sanitiser in food processing and handling applications. Commonly used chlorine compounds include: liquid chlorine, hypochlorites, inorganic chloramines, and organic chloramines. Chlorine-based sanitisers form hypochlorous acid (HOCl, the most active form) in solution. Available chlorine (the amount of HOCl present) is a function of pH. At pH 5, nearly all is in the form of HOCl. At pH 7.0, approximately 75% is HOCl. The maximumallowable level for no-rinse applications is 200ppm available chlorine, but recommended usage levels vary.

For hypochlorites, an exposure time of 1 min at a minimum concentration of 50ppm and a temperature of 24°C (75°F) is recommended. For each 10°C (18°F) drop in temperature, a doubling of exposure time is recommended. For chloramines, 200ppm for 1 min is recommended. Chlorine compounds are broad spectrum germicides which act on microbial membranes, inhibit cellular enzymes involved in glucose metabolism, have a lethal effect on DNA, and oxidise cellular protein.

Chlorine has activity at low temperature, is relatively cheap, and leaves minimal residue or film on surfaces. The activity of chlorine is dramatically affected by such factors as pH, temperature, and organic load. However, chlorine is less affected by water hardness when compared to other sanitisers. The major disadvantage to chlorine compound is corrosiveness to many metal surfaces. Health and safety concerns can occur due to skin irritation and mucous membrane damage in confined areas.

At low pH (below 4.0), deadly Cl_2 (mustard gas) can form. In recent years, concerns have also been raised about the use of chlorine as a drinking water disinfectant and as an antimicrobial with direct food contact (meat, poultry and shellfish). This concern is based upon the involvement of chlorine in the formation of potentially carcinogenic trihalomethanes (THMs) under appropriate conditions. While chlorine's benefits as a sanitiser far outweigh these risks, it is under scrutiny.

Chlorine dioxide (ClO_2) is currently being considered as a replacement for chlorine, since it appears to be more environmentally friendly. Stabilised ClO_2 has FDA approval for most applications in sanitising equipment or for use as a foam for environmental and non-food contact surfaces. Approval has also been granted for use in flume waters in fruits and vegetable operations and in poultry process waters. ClO_2 has 2.5 times the oxidising power of chlorine and, thus, less chemical is required.

Typical use concentrations range from 1to 10ppm. ClO_2's primary disadvantages are worker safety and toxicity. Its highly concentrated gases can be explosive and exposure risks to workers is higher thanthat for chlorine. Its rapid decomposition in the presence of light, or at temperatures greater than 50°C (122°F) makes on-site generation a recommended practice. Use of iodine as an antimicrobial agents dates back to the 1800s.

This sanitiser exists in many forms and usually exists with a surfactant as a carrier. These mixtures are termed iodophors. The most active agent is the dissociated free iodine. This form is most prevalent at low pH. The amount of dissociation from the surfactant is dependent upon the type of surfactant. Iodine solubility is very limited in water.

Generally recommended usage for iodophors is 12.5 to 25ppm for 1 min. It is generally thought that the bactericidal activity of iodine is through direct halogenation of proteins. More recent theories have centered upon cell wall damage and destruction of microbial enzyme activity. Iodophors, like chlorine compounds, have a very broad spectrum: being active against bacteria, viruses, yeasts, molds, fungi, and protozoans.

Iodine is highly temperature-dependent and vaporizes at 120°F. Thus, it is limited to lower temperature applications. The degree to which iodophors are affected by environmental factors is highly dependant upon properties of the surfactant used in the formulation. Iodophors are generally less affected by organic matter and water hardness than chlorine. However, loss of activity is pronounced at high pH. Iodine has a long history of use in wound treatment.

Since Quaternary Ammonium Compounds (QACs) are positively charged cations, their mode of action is related to their attraction to negatively charged materials such as bacterial proteins. It is generally accepted that the mode of action is at the membrane function. The carbon length of R-group side chain is, generally, directly related with sanitiser activity in QACs. However, because of the lower solubility in QACs composed of large carbon chains, these sanitisers may have lower activity than short chain structures. QACs are active and stable over a broad temperature range. Because they are surfactants, they possess some detergency. Thus, they are less affected by light soil than are other sanitisers.

However, heavy soil dramatically decreases activity. QACs generally have higher activity at alkaline pH. While lack of tolerance to hard water is often listed as a major disadvantage of QACs when compared to chlorine, some QACs are fairly tolerant of hard water. Activity can be improved by the use of EDTA as a chelator. QACs are effective against bacteria, yeasts, mold, and viruses. An advantage of QACs in some applications is that they leave a residual antimicrobial film. However, this would be a disadvantage in operations such as cultured dairy products, cheese, beer, etc. where microbial starter cultures are used.

QACs are generally more active against gram positive than gram negative bacteria. They are not highly effective against bacteriophages. Their incompatibility with certain detergents makes thorough rinsing following cleaning operations imperative.Further, many QAC formulations can cause foaming problems in CIP applications. Under recommended usage and precautions, QACs pose little toxicity or safety risks. Thus, they are in common use as environmental fogs and as room deodorisers.

However, care should be exercised in handling concentrated solutions or use as environmental fogging agents. Like QACs, acid-anionic sanitisers are surface-active sanitisers. These formulations include an inorganic acid plus a surfactant, and are often used for the dual function of acid rinse and sanitisation. Whereas QACs are positively charged, these sanitisers are negatively charged. Their activity is moderately affected by water hardness. Their low use pH, detergency, stability, low odor potential, and non-corrosiveness makes them highly desirable in some applications.

Fatty acid or carboxylic acid sanitisers were developed in the 1980s. Typical formulations include fatty acids plus other acids (phosphoric acids, organic acids). These agents also have the dual function of acid rinse and sanitisation. The major advantage over acid anionics is lower foaming potential. These sanitisers have a broad range of activity, are highly stable in dilute form, are stable to organic matter, and are stable to high temperature applications. These sanitisers have low activity above pH 3.5 - 4.0, are not very effective against yeasts and molds, and some formulations lose activity at temperatures below 10°C (50°F).

Peroxides or peroxy compounds contain at least one pair of covalently bonded oxygen atoms (-O-O-)and are divided into two groups: the inorganic group, containing hydrogen peroxide (HP) and related compounds; and the organic group, containing peroxyacetic acid (PAA) and related compounds. The primary mode of action for HP is through creating an oxidising environment and generation of singlet or superoxide oxygen (SO).

HP is fairly broad spectrum with slightly higher activity against gram-negative than gram-positive organisms. High concentrations of HP (5% and above) can be an eye and skin irritant. Thus, high concentrations should be handled with care. Peroxyacetic Acid (PAA) has been known for its germicidal properties for a long time. However, it has only found food-industry application in recent years and is being promoted as a potential chlorine replacement.

PAA is relatively stable at use strengths of 100 to 200ppm. Other desirable properties include: absence of foam and phosphates, low corrosiveness, tolerance to hard water, and favorable biodegradability. PAA solutions have been shown to be useful in removing biofilms. While precise mode of action mechanisms have not been determined, it is generally theorised that the PAA reaction with microorganisms is similar to that of HP. PAA, however, is highly active against both gram- positive and gram-negative microorganisms. The germicidal activity of PAA is dramatically affected by pH. Any pH increase above 7-8 drastically reduces the activity. PAA has a pungent odor and the concentrated product (40%) is a highly toxic, potent irritant, and powerful oxidiser. Thus, care must be used in its use.

Restroom Cleaning

Today's marketplace of custodial equipment affords housekeeping managers many advantages in cleaning restrooms, compared with the days of the traditional mop, bucket and wringer. The traditional method, though still in use, is increasingly falling behind the new technologies. Some new systems are simple, while others are more complex, but most systems enhance the performance of cleaning chemicals - if, in fact, any chemicals are used at all - and all while enabling managers to minimise complaints by effectively cleaning restrooms.

Vapour Cleaning systems are becoming increasingly popular. The systems use no chemicals. Instead, they use a tank that superheats the water, and operators spray the resulting steam onto the dirty areas with a special wand that features an applicator to which cleaning towels might be attached. The operator wipes all surfaces with the superheated vapor, changing the cloth as it becomes soiled. The units also have special heads that allow for crevice cleaning.

In addition to using these units for cleaning restrooms, cleaning crews also can use them for cleaning kitchens because the steam easily breaks down the grease. Also, when using the wand and towel attachment, the units might be effective in cleaning dirt off walls. Manufacturers of some of these systems claim that the units require no chemicals, but housekeeping managers should familiarise themselves with the claims and the infection-control needs of their facility.

Also, operators need to be aware that the vapor is hot and that handles of some wands might become hot. As a result, they will need to wear appropriate personal protective equipment. Several manufacturers now market restroom cleaning kits that might include a cleaning cart, a bucket and a series of extension handles with associated specialised mop heads and attachments. The cart has space for storing cleaning supplies and paper products. Increasingly, crews are replacing old cotton-string mops with microfiber flat mops that are easier to use, lighter and enable aggressive cleaning of the surface. The restroom cleaning kits give the person cleaning restrooms all of the necessary products they might need on the job site.

Some advocates of microfiber cleaning cloths say that the cloths eliminate or mitigate the need for cleaning chemicals. Realistically, crews often can enhance their cleaning efforts in restrooms by applying the appropriate chemicals during the cleaning process. Specialised power washers for cleaning restrooms have been available for several years now.

Generally, the power washer is cart-mounted for carrying limited cleaning supplies and might come in various sizes. Basically, after the floor has been swept, the unit allows the operator to power-wash the restroom from ceiling to floor and to air dry the room before use. These units have specialised chemicals, applied through a solution pick-up hose, that afford deep cleaning and drying of surfaces without leaving spots, much like an effective dishwashing agent.

More advanced units not only can allow an operator to power spray a room but can also pick up the residue solution after cleaning to minimise the time that a restroom is out of service. When using these units, operators need use all appropriate safety precautions. For example, crews should not spray chemicals into electrical outlets, and they should make sure that paper goods are adequately protected from solution overspray.

When used correctly, these units really do deliver deep cleaning to restrooms. Manufacturers have provided a new generation of equipment for housekeeping managers to specify to improve the level of restroom cleaning in their facilities. Several can help minimise the use of chemicals. Housekeeping managers who want to curtail complaints concerning their facilities' restrooms and minimise the impact of cleaning chemicals and processes on the environment have more options than ever today. They can achieve these goals by learning about those options. Today's environmentally friendly chemicals and equipment are increasingly cost competitive, have increased efficacy, limit damage to the environment and minimise costs to an organisation for disposal of chemicals.

The proper maintenance of a health care facility increases the awareness of other employees of the necessity of good sanitary practices. Good housekeeping practices increase moral and public relations. No one wants to work in an area that smells or is dirty. Sanitation depends upon cleaning thoroughness. There should be procedures in writing to fit each area of the facility such as walls, floors, windows, beds, furniture, draperies, carpets, waste containers, bathrooms, equipment, stairs, elevators, special-care equipment and handling of infectious waste for disposal.

Role of Cleaning Workers

Maids and housekeeping cleaners perform any combination of light cleaning duties to maintain private households or commercial establishments, such as hotels, restaurants, and hospitals, clean and orderly. In hotels, aside from cleaning and maintaining the premises, maids and housekeeping cleaners may deliver ironing boards, cribs, and rollaway beds to guests' rooms. In hospitals, they also may wash bedframes, brush mattresses, make beds, and disinfect and sterilise equipment and supplies with germicides and sterilising equipment.

Janitors, maids, and cleaners use various equipment, tools, and cleaning materials. For one job they may need a mop and bucket, for another an electric polishing machine and a special cleaning solution. Improved building materials, chemical cleaners, and power equipment have made many tasks easier and less time consuming, but cleaning workers must learn the proper use of equipment and cleaners to avoid harming floors, fixtures, and themselves. Cleaning supervisors coordinate, schedule, and supervise the activities of janitors and cleaners.

They assign tasks and inspect building areas to see that work has been done properly, issue supplies and equipment, and inventory stocks to ensure that an adequate amount of supplies is present. They also screen and hire job applicants, train new and experienced employees, and recommend promotions, transfers, or dismissals.

Supervisors may prepare reports concerning the occupancy of rooms, hours worked, and department expenses. Some also perform cleaning duties. Cleaners and servants in private households dust and polish furniture; sweep, mop, and wax floors; vacuum; and clean ovens, refrigerators, and bathrooms. They also may wash dishes, polish silver, and change and make beds. Some wash, fold, and iron clothes; a few wash windows.

Supervisors conduct inspections to ensure that the building is cleaned properly and the team is functioning efficiently. Building cleaning workers usually work inside heated, well-lighted buildings. However, they sometimes work outdoors, sweeping walkways, mowing lawns, or shoveling snow. Working with machines can be noisy, and some tasks, such as cleaning bathrooms and trash rooms, can be dirty and unpleasant. Janitors may suffer cuts, bruises, and burns from machines, handtools, and chemicals. They spend most of their time on their feet, sometimes lifting or pushing heavy furniture or equipment.

Janitors and cleaners work in nearly every type of establishment and held about 2.3 million jobs. They accounted for about 57 percent of all building cleaning workers. About 28 percent worked for firms supplying building maintenance services on a contract basis, 21 percent were employed in educational institutions, and 2 percent worked in hotels. Other employers included hospitals, restaurants, religious institutions, manufacturing firms, government agencies, and operators of apartment buildings, office buildings, and other types of real estate.

Maids and housekeepers held about 1.5 million jobs. Hotels, motels, and other traveler accommodations employed the most maids and housekeepers-27 percent-while private households employed the second most: 25 percent. Eight percent were employed in hospitals; and, a similar percentage worked in nursing and other residential care facilities.

Most building cleaners learn their skills on the job. Usually, beginners work with an experienced cleaner, doing routine cleaning. As they gain more experience, they are assigned more complicated tasks. In some cities, programs run by unions, government agencies, or employers teach janitorial skills. Students learn how to clean buildings thoroughly and efficiently, how to select and safely use various cleansing agents, and how to operate and maintain machines, such as wet and dry vacuums, buffers, and polishers.

Dish Washing

Maybe you've never seen what happens to a sinkful of dishes left to sit, but it isn't pretty. Smells, stains, and odd fungal growth usually go with forgotten dirty dishes. Cleaning dishes daily is the best choice all around.

Tools for dish washing:

Dishpans: If you don't have a double sink, a dishpan can be used to rinse or hold your dishes during the washing process. Choose one that is a good size, but remember if it's too big, it will make filling and emptying the pan a messy difficult process.

Dishrack: Dishracks prevent water from collecting and pooling in your newly clean dishes. They prevent bacteria growth and help protect dishes from banging into one another. Many models now have fold down prongs for easier storage when the dishes are done. Choose a dishrack with a sloping bottom mat to allow water to easily drain off into a sink.

Dish Towels: Dish towels will be necessary to buff out spots and dry still wet dishes. Remember to make the rinsing water as hot as possible to allow the dishes to quickly airdry. Airdrying is more sanitary than cloth drying. Dish towels pick up bacteria that is then transferred to every dish dried. Always use clean dishcloths to dry dishes. Lint-free cloths may be needed for silverware.

Mats: A rubber mat placed in the bottom of the sink helps prevent breakage when dishes are loaded and moved around.

Scrapers, scrubbers, and sponges: Steel wool pads, plastic scrubbers, and double sided sponges may all be useful during dishwashing. Throw away steel wool pads and scrubbers when they show excessive signs of wear. Allow sponges to air dry after use.

Rubber Gloves: Rubber gloves increase handling power and protect hands. Find a good pair of rubber gloves, disposable gloves, or latex free gloves and protect your hands.

Dishcloths: As with sponges, dishcloths must not be allowed to sit for long periods of time in dishwater. Remember to launder your dishcloths frequently to prevent bacteria, staining, and odors.

Dishliquids: Dish liquids come in many scents, specialties, and varieties. Be sure not to add too much, which only makes washing and rinsing dishes more difficult. Check out some environmentally friendly options.

Laundry Washing

Not every family needs to wash laundry daily, but many of us find that at least a daily load of laundry is necessary. A daily load can help prevent a mad dash to find a baseball jersey in the bottom of a hamper.

Stain Removal

Removing stains can sometimes seem like a complex algebra problem. By the time you determine the stain type, origin of the stain, fabric type and color schemed you can feel pessimistic about stain removal. Try these 10 simple stain removal rules to get your laundry in shape.

1. *Act quickly.*

Fresh stains make stain removal an easy task. Give yourself the upper hand by treating stains as promptly after they happen as possible. If your stains are on a non-washable fabric, take them to the dry cleaners as soon as possible. Be sure to point out the stain to the dry cleaner and describe the nature of the stain. This makes the likelihood of stain removal success greater.

2. *Follow the directions.*

Follow the directions on any stain removal products you

use. Don't forget to follow washing directions on the stained clothes.

3. Test in a hidden area.

Don't forget to test any stain removal methods on a hidden seam or other inconspicous spot. You want to check for colorfastness before applying a treatment to a large or noticeable area of the clothing. Do not use if the color changes.

4.Remove stains from the back.

Place the stained garment with the stain upside down on top of a clean white cloth. Apply stain treatment to the back of the stain. Our goal is to remove the stain from the clothing instead of making it travel all the way through to the other side. Make sure to move the stained clothing to a fresh spot as the stain begins to remove itself from the clothing and onto the cloth.

5. Be careful with dry cleaning solvents.

Make sure to rinse thoroughly, and allow to air dry any garment that's had dry cleaning solvents used on it. These solvents can be a fire hazard in a washing machine. Remember never to put dry cleaning solvents directly into the washing machine.

6. Be wary of even color removal with bleach.

Bleaching only one stained spot on a garment may result in uneven color removal for the entire garment. Consider using the appropriate bleach listed in the garment tag to bleach the entire garment.

7. Don't mix stain removal products.

Mixing different chemicals can cause toxic odors and mixed results on your clothing.

8. Wash stain treated items.

Remember to thoroughly wash items that have treated with stain removal products to remove product residue and also the stain residue.

9. Be patient.

Stain removal can take time. Sometimes repeat treatments may be required. Be sure to thoroughly check the garment before drying to determine if a repeat treatment is necessary. Drying will cause a stain to set.

10. Some stains won't leave.

For some stains, no stain removal idea or tip can get rid of them without damaging the clothing or its color. But take heart in the fact that the other 9 general stain removal tips will give you a fighting chance against all the stains in your laundry basket. Just a few simple guidelines can take the guesswork out of stain removal.

Sorting

Sorting is the easiest part of washing clothes, right? Wrong. Sorting is the most difficult and time consuming part of laundry. If done incorrectly sorting ruins clothes and can damage machines. When done properly sorting saves invaluable time, energy, and money. There are 6 main things to look for when sorting laundry. Actually placing the clothing in the proper pile is only one of them.

1. Check clothing tags.

Read the tags thoroughly to determine how the clothes should be washed dried and ironed. Most items will have mainly normal washing instructions. You might be surprised though that you have items that are meant to be hand washed or not dried in the drier. Set these items aside in their own "Special Care" pile. Check here for Fabric Link's guide to Fabric Care Symbols.

2. Turn clothing right side out.

Make sure none of the legs of your pants, or arms of your shirts are stuck in the garment improperly. If you are washing overalls, take the time now to clasp the latches of the overalls to their proper buttons, keeping them from getting broken, stretched or ripped. If you had any clothing tags that instructed you to wash the clothing inside out, make sure you remembered to do so.

3. Check all pockets.

It's best to have a bowl nearby to hold the contents of your pockets. Failing to check pockets can leave some nasty surprises.

4. Check for sewing repairs.

Make sure there aren't any loose threads, rips, button repairs, or other sewing repairs. If you find any, repair them before you wash the clothes. Washing them with problems will only make the problems bigger.

5. Check for stains

They will need to be pretreated or soaked before washing and drying. If you dry a stain, you'll most likely have a stain for life.

6. Sort the clothing.

There are many different methods to sorting. Some people sort by color. Others sort by fabric type. There are some adventurous souls who actually never sort clothing. Your sorting method will likely be determined by the size of your family and contents of your wardrobes. Here are some of the sorting categories that may demand special attention.

Whites- Whites go separate because we want them to stay white. One red sock that isn't colorfast can turn an entire white load pink. More often than not whites need a warmer water temperature than other clothing to ensure proper cleaning.

Reds and or Bright Colors- Colorfast pinks, purples, reds, and oranges can be mixed together to make a full load.

Some people like to sort everything else into its color category to get a nice mix of small and large items for each load. For example, with a large family you may end up with a blue load, green load, khaki load, black load, etc. If your items are colorfast, (most clothing will be) you can combine colors together.

Sanitation Practices and Procedures

Water

— Drinking water used by the Laboratory shall be tested routinely by the Plant Maintenance and Engineering Section to ensure uniform and proper consistency and compliance with all federal, state, or local sanitation requirements for both chemical and biological contaminants.

— The drinking water supply shall not contain impurities in concentrations which may be hazardous to the health of the consumer or which would cause offense to the sense of sight, taste or smell.

— The drinking water supply system shall be installed according to the National Plumbing Code and all other federal, state, and local plumbing requirements and shall be maintained in good condition.

— The drinking water system must be protected against backflow with connections and plumbing devices approved by the American National Standards Institute (ANSI).

— An adequate supply of potable water shall be available within a reasonable distance to any location at which employees are regularly engaged in work. Under certain conditions this requirement may be met by approved bottled water dispensers. These dispensers shall be designed, constructed, and serviced so that sanitary conditions are maintained and shall be capable of being closed.

— All water lines shall be distinctly marked according to the type of water flowing through them. Outlets for non-potable water, such as deionized water, distilled water, etc., shall be labeled to indicated that the water is not to be used for drinking, washing, or cooking purposes.

Food

— All foods and beverages shall be prepared, stored, displayed, dispensed, placed, or served in a way that they are protected from dust, flies, vermin, pollution by rodents, unnecessary handling, airborne droplet infection, overhead leakage, or other contamination to ensure compliance with all federal, state, and local requirements.

— Refrigerators located throughout PPPL must be labeled as to their contents with signs such as "FOOD ONLY" or "CHEMICALS ONLY." Refrigerators labeled for "FOOD ONLY" shall not be used to store non-food substances. Food shall not be consumed or stored where toxic or chemical materials are handled or stored.

— Microwaves used for food preparation are to be maintained in a sanitary condition at all times. Periodic inspection of microwave ovens is conducted by Safety Office personnel.

— All suspected or alleged cases of food poisoning must be reported to the Dispensary.

Waste

— All sanitary sewage shall be released from Laboratory controlled areas into sanitary sewer lines.

— Drainage through storm sewers and drainage ditches must conform with the water quality standards of the New Jersey Department of Environmental Protection.

— All chemicals and substances which are toxic, reactive, corrosive or flammable shall not be released into the sanitary or storm sewer system.

— All garbage and trash shall be accumulated outside of buildings in closed containers and shall be removed promptly from the premises.

— Items which are required to be recycled or are earmarked for scrap or special disposal shall be placed in designated containers.

Toilet and Locker Facilities

Adequate toilets, washrooms, lockers, and other essential sanitary facilities shall be readily accessible for employees near their work areas. These facilities shall be maintained in a clean and sanitary condition. Soap in a dispenser and hand drying apparatus shall be provided at each wash location.

Pest, Weed, and Animal Control

— A continuous programme of insect and rodent abatement administered by Plant Maintenance and Enginnering shall be maintained.

— All pesticides, including those for use by contractors, shall be reviewed by the Safety Office for health and environmental impacts prior to use.

— Animal Control actions shall be initiated through Plant.

Maintenance and Engineering and shall be conducted humanely under appropriate local humane requirements.

— All herbicides or other chemicals used for grounds maintenance, including those for use by contractors, shall be reviewed by the Safety Office for health and environmental impacts prior to use.

All buildings shall be kept clean and orderly with:

1. Floors free of spilled liquids, debris,and clutter.
2. Light fixtures and windows clean.
3. Walls well-painted.
4. Machinery and equipment kept neat and in order. 5. Aisles clearly marked and kept free, with materials properly stacked in designated areas.

The floor of every workroom shall be maintained, so far as is practicable, in a dry condition. Where wet processes are used, drainage shall be maintained and false floors, platforms, mats, or other dry standing shall be provided where practicable, or appropriate waterproof and slip resistant foot gear shall be provided. To facilitate cleaning, every floor, working place, and passageway shall be kept free from protruding nails, splinters, loose boards, and unnecessary holes and openings.

An adequate supply of well-constructed, closed containers for trash, recycling materials, scrap, etc. shall be provided and emptied on a frequent basis.Aisles, doorways, and stairways shall be adequate for emergency escape, shall be plainly marked, and unblocked. Exits and emergency equipment, such as fire extinguishers, eyewashes, etc., shall be properly identified and readily accessible.

Procedures for periodic review to ensure the proper and prompt disposal of obsolete stock, parts, and waste shall be used. Excess chemicals, especially those for which a use is not foreseeable within the next six months, should be disposed of through the Hazardous Materials Section.

Sanitation and Health

In addition to facility, food, and water cleanliness, personal cleanliness is essential to maintain a healthful work environment. Inflammation of the skin (dermatitis) is an ever-present problem in an industrial or laboratory setting. Adequate washing and prevention of contact with agents harmful to the skin are the most effective measures of skin care.

— Wear clean clothing. Change clothing that has been contaminated with materials which may be harmful. Use disposable clothing as necessary.

— Use the proper personal protective equipment such as chemical gloves, face shields, aprons, etc.

— For minor exposures to relatively inert materials that cause excessive soiling, hand-protective creams may be applied before the job is started.

— Thoroughly wash after any job that causes excessive soiling of the skin and particularly after contact with agents harmful to the skin. Use hand-cleansing creams —not acetone, mineral spirits, and other such solvents —to remove greases, dyes, carbon, paints, resins, or other adhering materials. Hand cleansing creams do an excellent job and are available from stock.

— Solvent use can cause irritation of the skin. After excessive washing and contact with cleaning solutions and agents, handconditioning creams should be used to replace oil in the skin.

— Emergency showers and eyewashes are for emergency use to dilute and wash away contaminants in those critical seconds right after an accident in which you may be sprayed or splashed with a chemical. Employees should know the location of and how to use the emergency equipment nearest their work areas. Emergency showers and eyewashes are checked periodically by Plant Maintenance and Engineering. Emergency eyewashes should be flushed at a minimum of once per month.

Waste Prevention

Waste prevention is a win-win approach that is neither costly nor cumbersome. It is also the approach that tops the list of solid waste management options adopted by the US Environmental Protection Agency, followed by (in order of desirability) recycling (including composting), incineration, and landfill disposal. Unlike all the other strategies, waste prevention decreases the amount (and toxicity) of waste generated.

Prevention also reduces the cost of collection, recycling, and disposal systems, and it helps alleviate the political conflicts that often surround waste management systems. The growth of recycling during the 1980s and

1990s represents a step forward in the management of materials, because recycling mines the waste stream for valuable materials that can be reprocessed into new products. But waste prevention—including the reuse of products—is even more basic. It avoids the creation of waste in the first place.

Solid Waste

In recent years, waste as the visible result of the inefficient use of natural resources. Products and packages with short life cycles (including those considered "disposable") create problems that go far beyond disposal. Short-lived products also contribute to the depletion of natural resources and to the creation of pollution during materials extraction, product manufacture, and product use. Once discarded, products and packaging impose substantial environmental and economic burdens on the nation.

Solutions for Waste Prevention

Simply defined, waste prevention is a reduction in the amount and/or toxicity of materials entering the waste stream prior to recycling, treatment, or disposal. "Source reduction"—that is, reducing waste at the source—is another term for this approach. Waste prevention can be part of an "environmentally sustainable" way of living and doing business meaning it can be sustained long-term in harmony with the environment, without depleting limited resources and without polluting our air, land, or water.

Waste prevention is a winning strategy, both environmentally and economically. It can be accomplished in a variety of ways. Waste prevention may mean a change in practices to encourage the use of durable, repairable, and reusable products. It may mean changing a product or package to reduce the materials needed to make that product or package. Or it may even mean eliminating the need for a specific product or certain packaging elements.

Strategies that prevent waste also conserve valuable resources. For example, reusing corrugated boxes—the largest-volume component of a hotel's waste stream—reduces raw material use, avoids the need for energy to manufacture or recycle boxes, and prevents the pollution that arises from the manufacture and recycling of additional boxes. Waste prevention is a call to do more with less. Making this transition will require:

- Fundamental changes in the design and use of products and packages and in systems for distributing them
- Essential shifts in business, institutional, and individual practices to achieve more efficient materials use
- Public and private promotion of waste reduction and careful resource use by communities and businesses.

It is difficult to estimate the amount of solid waste generated by individual hotels. However, critical factors include the number of employees, the number of guest rooms, the scope of kitchen and restaurant services, and the size and number of meeting rooms or convention facilities. Luxury hotels usually employ more staff and offer more services to guests than more moderately priced properties, and thus often generate more waste. Two categories of garbage dominate the typical hotel waste stream: paper and food/organics.

Starting a comprehensive waste prevention programme is a team effort, It requires planning, communication with all employees and departments, and the development of well-understood goals. To get started, hotels and motels can target their waste prevention initiatives by looking in three key directions:

— Assessing purchasing decisions
— Understanding how materials and equipment are used
— Examining the waste stream.

Assessing purchasing decisions: Since most products purchased eventually end up in the hotel's waste stream, a purchasing assessment can determine if longer-lasting, repairable, and reusable items could replace shorter-lived, non-repairable, single-use products. Purchasing plays an especially important role in waste prevention. Simply, if an item is not bought, it cannot be thrown away. Incorporating waste prevention objectives into purchasing policies can decrease the amount of waste generated, encourage vendors to develop and sell products that create less waste, and often save money. Keep in mind that hotels—like other businesses—pay for the use of items twice: once upon purchase and again at disposal.

To explore the role purchasing can play in waste prevention, each purchasing agent or general manager could begin by asking, for each item delivered, why do we have this? If an item is not deemed essential, why buy it? If it is needed, does the product chosen make the most economical use of materials and offer the least possible toxicity? Do vendors sell less harmful alternatives? Can the property buy the product in bulk to reduce costs and packaging waste? Buying products in the largest quantity possible in one package utilises less packaging per ounce than several smaller containers. Can containers be returned for reuse, or can they be recycled?

Understanding how materials and equipment are used: Besides procurement, hotels can prevent waste by changing the way they use products and materials. For example, circulating a memo to five people instead of distributing separate copies to each person saves four copies; using electronic mail saves six copies, including the original. Hotels can also "intensify" their use of products to keep them in working condition longer and to get the maximum use out of a product.

For instance, by repairing broken guest room furniture, office equipment, and kitchen appliances, hotels can lengthen the useful life of these products, keeping them out of the waste stream longer and saving money, too. In addition, hotels can reuse materials from one area in other parts of the property—eliminating the need to buy, use, and dispose of additional items—or they can donate them to charity.

Examining the waste stream: The goal of examining a property's waste stream is to look for opportunities to prevent waste by identifying materials that are:

— Major components of the waste stream (for example, office paper)

— Easy to reduce (for example, by composting landscaping waste)

— Sources of pollution in the local waste management system (for example, batteries).

To learn what materials make up a hotel's waste stream—and the cost of handling them—a hotel could undertake any or all of the following activities:

— A visual inspection of the hotel, conducted by walking through various parts of the property, including guest rooms, food service areas, offices, and loading docks

— Interviews with staff in each area, including grounds crews, housekeeping staff, office personnel, and food service workers

— Examination of purchasing records

— Sorting of waste by department (or hotel-wide); in "dumpster diving," "divers" physically separate and measure materials discarded in dumpsters and recycling bins

— An examination of waste hauling records to learn the weight or volume of waste generated and the cost of disposing of or recycling that waste By gathering quantitative information on discarded materials, hotels can set realistic goals for preventing waste.

Balancing waste prevention with service and ratings. Waste prevention does not have to mean a reduction in the level of service offered, even for the most luxurious hotel. In many cases, waste prevention can be an "invisible" strategy, one that takes place behind the scenes of a hotel's public operations. However, other strategies may be more visible—for example, using refillable shampoo dispensers instead of mini-sized bottles—and managers may be concerned that their guests will perceive the change as a cut in service. Yet there are many ways to make guests feel pampered without contributing to the waste stream.

Some luxury hotels have been able to use the money saved by purchasing refillable or reusable products to offer higher quality products overall, such as betterquality shampoos in the refillable dispensers. Hotels might offer guests a glass of champagne upon arrival, fresh flowers in the room, or a basket of fruit. Managers may also be concerned that some waste prevention measures could lower the ratings the property receives from independent travel organisations. According to representatives of Mobil Travel Guide and the American Automobile Association's (AAA) Industry Evaluations department—the two leading sources of these ratings—this is not necessarily the case.

Hotel evaluations are based on the overall level of service a property provides, so presentation counts, along with the specific items presented. At the same time, hotel inspectors may evaluate certain changes as a cut in service—regardless of their presentation. Representatives of AAA point out that hotel managers can contact their inspectors to discuss the implementation of waste prevention measures at their properties.

Mobil Travel Guide does not rely on a checklist or set criteria regarding the specific nature of the items or services a hotel must supply in order to be awarded a top rating. A marketing approach. Indeed, some hotels have found that their guests appreciate those steps taken to help the environment. Educating guests about a hotel or motel's policies and asking for feedback can be an important part of a hotel's marketing approach.

Guests who have become used to "green" habits in their own homes may appreciate a door-hanger that allows them to decide whether or not to have newspapers delivered or sheets changed daily throughout their visit. Properties that cater especially to families might choose to educate and involve their guests in waste prevention, while businessoriented properties might opt for a more subtle approach. Individual managers can determine how to balance waste prevention with the level of convenience and comfort their guests have come to expect.

Waste Prevention Strategies in Hotel and Motel

Within a hotel or motel, each functional area presents its own set of waste prevention challenges. The list below, which suggests a variety of specific strategies for preventing waste, is organised according to these functional areas.

Guest rooms

— Review policies for guest room amenities and the packaging of those items. Inform guests of efforts to provide amenities that have less impact on the environment.

— Provide soap, shampoo, and lotion in refillable dispensers, instead of individual containers. Provide individual containers only upon request.

— Do not remove "gift" amenities from the room after a guest departs unless the seal on the package is broken. Leave unopened amenities in the room for the next guest.

— Reduce size of individually packaged items, such as bar soap, to reduce the quantities left over.

— Rather than offering individually packaged amenities, consider offering another type of gift, such as a basket of fruit or a bottle of wine.

— Wait to replace-half-filled toilet paper rolls and tissue boxes until they are almost completely used. Leave new rolls and tissue boxes in bathrooms for guests to replace.

— If half-used items must be removed, place them in employee rest rooms or donate them to charity.

— Give newpapers, shoeshine kits, and showercaps to guests only upon request. To avoid delivering newspapers to guests who don't want them, provide guests with a door hanger that allows them to request the next morning's papers.

— Deliver newspapers to guest rooms without plastic bag wrappings.

— Provide guest rooms with unwrapped, reusable drinking glasses and coffee cups. Check with the local health department about storing glasses upside down on trays, rather than using disposable paper covers.

— Eliminate the use of plastic liners in ice buckets.

— Eliminate the use of paper doilies and paper tray covers,

— Reduce printed information placed in rooms.

Condense printed material where possible or designate a special television channel for hotel information.

— Order only as many telephone directories as the number of rooms and phones. Directory distributors often deliver many more copies than are needed.

Laundry and Housekeeping

1. *Laundry and Dry Cleaning*

   — Ask guests whether they would like to have their towels and sheets replaced daily, or whether they want to "help the environment" by reusing them. Besides saving water and energy, reduced laundering will also reduce the use of detergent and bleach. Make sure guest bathrooms have enough towel-rail space to hang wet towels.

   — After dry cleaning, return clothes in reusable garment bags to eliminate the need for single-use plastic bags.

   — Offer plastic wrap for dry cleaned clothing only upon request.

   — Eliminate cardboard backing for laundered shirts.

   — Reuse wire clothes hangers from guest drycleaning services for guest bathrobes and employee uniforms or return them to vendors.

2. *Resing Textiles*

   — Convert damaged textiles, such as uniforms and linens, into useful items. For example, it's possible to turn torn bed sheets, towels, and banquet linens into reusable guest-room laundry bags, baby bibs, crib bumper pads, aprons, cleaning rags, and bar covers. Another possibility: repair torn bed linen and reuse it on smaller cots or cribs.

— Replace single-use items with reusable items such as napkins, tablecloths, and hand towels. When they are worn, turn them into cleaning rags.

— Dye stained towels a darker color for reuse at the pool or beach, or as cleaning cloths.

— Extend the useful life of draperies by, rotating them to expose different portions to sunlight.

3. *Cleaning Products*

— Buy cleaning products in bulk and in concentrated form, because one large container of product uses less packaging per ounce than several smaller containers. At the same time, order only what can be used before the product expires.

— Install mixing stations in the housekeeping department to reduce spillage. Educate staff on proper mixing of concentrates to avoid waste and save money.

— Fill smaller reusable containers with cleaning products from larger containers.

— Use refillable pump spray bottles that can be reused instead of single-use aerosol cans.

— Buy cleaning products that are biodegradable.

— Buy supplies from vendors who take back the containers in which they ship cleaning materials

— Clean and reuse dustmop heads.

— Use reusable vacuum cleaner bags.

4. *Reducing the Use of Toxic Chemicals*

— Minimise the use of products that contain toxic chemicals. The types of products that may pose toxic risks include pesticides, herbicides, bleaches, oven cleaners, drain cleaners, acids, disinfectants, general cleaning chemicals, caustic cleaners, window cleaners, solvents, paints, adhesives, fuels, oils and grease, and hydraulic fluids. Begin by identifying where toxic chemicals are being used and the reason for their use. Review handling, storage, and disposal procedures and compile a record of toxic materials use. Where possible, identify, test, and use environmentally preferable alternatives.

— With the approval of the hotel's engineer, use a plunger or a snake rather than chemical solutions to remove plumbing obstructions, as long as the hotel's pipes are not in fragile condition. This avoids deleterious effects on waterways from the use of chemicals.

— Reduce the need for pesticide applications in guest rooms and employee work areas by making these areas less attractive to crawling pests. Remove food containers, garbage, and recycling containers frequently; clean employee break rooms daily; and report cracks around doors and windows to the engineering department.

— Check labels on room deodorizers for hazardous chemical content.

— Deodorizers are often used to mask smoke and mildew odors. Reduce the need for these products by: cleaning air conditioner coils and changing air conditioner filters regularly; sealing cracks around windows, doors, and air conditioning units; and operating air conditioners at temperatures recommended by the engineering department.

— Check buckets, cans, drums, and other chemical containers periodically and replace leaky ones.

— Use a containment pan at all times to prevent the leaching of unused chemicals, such as cleaning chemicals, oils, grease, and caustic cleaners.

— Clean chemical leaks and spills immediately.

— Store unused chemicals in a cool, dry, and well-ventilated place.

— Dispose of chemicals according to label instructions.

— Use rechargeable batteries wherever possible.

— Collect old alkaline, dry cell, and worn-out rechargeable batteries used in hotel walkie-talkies and pagers at a central collection point and dispose of them in accordance with local requirements. Many municipalities have special rules for disposing of batteries, and some locales have battery collection programmes. Batteries may contain toxic chemicals. If they are disposed of with other garbage, they may enter landfills, garbage incinerators, home septic systems, or public sewer systems. From there they can move into air, land, and water, where they may affect public health and the environment.

2

Kitchen Hygiene and Cleanliness

Hygiene and Cleanliness

It is easy to think that the clean kitchen is a hygienic one, but this does not necessarily followed. Cross contamination, poor temperature control, and many other dangerous practices can exist in the cleanest of kitchens, and many of the reported outbreaks arise from clean premises.

To go to extremes, an army field kitchen in a combat zone may be anything but clean, with mud floors, canvass walls and wooden trestles, yet, because of the type of food handled, and the way it is presented, it will still be hygienic. Cleanliness however is still very important. Among other reasons a high standard should be kept up to:

1. Provide a pleasant and attractive working environment.
2. Reduce the chance of a pest infestation building up without being noticed, or provide food for pests.
3. Allow disinfections procedures to work.
4. Prevent damage to, or reduction in efficiency of, equipment.
5. Foster efficient and economic working methods, with a minimum of waste.

6. Reduce risks of accident.
7. Promote a favorable image to the customer.

Cleanliness also has an additional vital importance in that staffs are unlikely to act in a hygienic way if their surroundings are dirty. In this respect cleaning cannot be divorced from hygiene, and while it is not all there is to hygiene, a clean kitchen provides a good start.

Personal Hygiene

The following is a list of basic requirements for every food worker:

1. Bath regularly, daily if possible. Keep your hair and finger nails clean and in good condition. Keep hair covered while at work
2. Keep your teeth clean and in good condition, otherwise your mouth will become the home for potentially dangerous germs. Visit the dentist regularly, not less than once every six months.
3. Wear clean clothes and the minimum of personal jewellery, watches and rings. If rings must be worn, they should be removed for washing hands.
4. Always wash your hands when first coming on duty, just before you start handling food, when you have used the W.C. or been in the toilet area, when you have handled raw meat before touching cooked foods, and when you have smoked or eaten anything, and when your hands are dirty.
5. Keep all sores, burns, cuts, spots and boils etc. covered with clean waterproof dressings. Report to your supervisor if wearing plasters interferes with your work. He/she may be able to arrange alternative duties.

6. Do not smoke, handle tobacco or any similar product, or spit in a food room. Do not cough or sneeze over food.
7. Report any illness to your supervisor/manager, when you become ill, without any delay. This applies even when on holiday, if possible, and on your days off. When visiting a doctor, always make sure that he/she knows that you are a food worker.
8. Avoid unnecessary handling of food. Hands are not sterile after washing.

Above all, use your common sense. If you think you, or the way you behave can contaminate food or otherwise cause danger, do something about it straight away.

Hand Care

Hands, more than anything else, are likely to contaminate foods unless great care is exercised. Washing hands properly is part of the care that will prevent contamination, but only part. Healthy skin is just as important so the points to keep in mind are listed here:

1. Keep hands dry as far as is possible, and dry your hands thoroughly after washing them or getting them wet. Do not leave them to air dry. Soap, even bactericidal soap, will not sterilize hands, but on dry healthy skin, most germs will not survive.
2. When washing your hands do it properly removing all traces of dirt. As well as causing a risk of contamination, dirt will irritate the skin and allow germs to flourish on it.
3. After using detergents or cleaning agents, rinse your hands. Thoroughly in clean running water until the "soapy" feel has gone, then dry them properly. Even small traces of detergents can irritate the skin, and it

is usually failure to rinse hands properly rather than the use of detergents that causes skin irritation.

4. If rubber gloves are used for any reason, make sure that the insides of the gloves are clean and dry before you put them on. Wash them after use, turn them inside out and leave to dry.
5. If any cleaner is used, where the instructions say that gloves should be worn, make sure that gloves are worn. Sometimes gloves will appear to be unnecessary and under normal conditions this might be so. The catering worker however is in a special position as regards the use of cleaning agents as it is repeated exposure over a long period of time that does the damage to skin, so gloves must be worn for this reason.
6. Keep cuts, scrapes and abrasions on the skin covered with clean and washable plasters and a finger stall if needed. If you have cuts etc. and the nature of your work both involves handling "sensitive" foods and makes the wearing of plasters difficult, see if your supervisor can arrange other work.
7. Keep fingernails trimmed, in good condition and clean at all times.
8. If you suffer from a rash or abnormal condition of the skin, see your doctor for advice and make sure that he/she knows you are a food worker. Report any such rash etc. to your supervisor.

The main thing to remember however is that healthy clean skin will kill off most germs that invade it. When the skin is broken, damaged, or dried out for whatever the cause, it becomes a home for germs. Skin care therefore is vital.

Cleaning & Detergents

Cleaning means, a process intended to remove unwanted

material of no value to a level that is visually acceptable, prevents the impairment of the function of an area or the equipment and fittings in it, and does not foster pests. It must also be to a level where chemical disinfections can be carried out satisfactorily, where needed, without being affected by the remaining material: (The unwanted material is generally called "dirt" or "soil".)

The process usually involves three stages, as follows:

a) The removal of gross, loose dirt by mechanical action.

b) The penetration of the film remaining by a combination of heat and chemicals, and its loosening and suspension.

c) The removal or rinsing off of loose suspended dirt.

The chemical normally used for the purpose of cleaning is called a detergent. All cleaning agents are in fact detergents, even soap, although detergents are generally taken to be synthetic liquid compounds, comprising of Surfactants, Alkaline builders, Water Softeners and a variety of other chemicals according to the use to which the detergent is put. Detergents can however come in a variety of forms from powders and gels to thick and thin liquids, of varying degrees of activity.

Nature of Dirt & Cleaning Processes

Dirt in the kitchen has different characteristics, which affect the way in which it can be removed. Forgetting loose dirt that can be swept off a surface there are two important classes.

1. Alkaline Soluble Dirt
2. Acid Soluble Dirt

Most cleaners in the kitchen are alkaline and are made to deal with fats, carbon deposits and food wastes) which can be dissolved by them as part of the chemical action.

A particular type of dirt found in the kitchen, scale, will however never is removed by an alkaline cleaner as it is acid soluble and for that an acid cleaner needs to be used. There is a third class of "dirt", that which is soluble in neither acid nor alkaline, most often found in kitchens as "stains". Adding either chemical type however strong will never remove this type of dirt and a solvent has to be used. As solvents are usually very specific in their action, it is usually better to get specialist advice on particular problems. Chemicals in any case are only part of the cleaning picture. The process of cleaning is best defined as:

The systematic application of energy to remove dirt. That energy can be supplied in three ways, or in combination as

1. *Mechanical energy*: scrubbing, rubbing, scraping etc.
2. *Chemical energy*: alkaline or acids.
3. *Heat*: hot water or dry heat as in an oven.

The particular form or combination of energy used will depend on the amount of dirt and how firmly it is attached to the surface, the situation and time available to do the job. Most importantly it will also depend on the nature of the surface to be cleaned, called the substrate, and whether it will be damaged by any of the forms. Cleaning therefore means the choosing of the type of energy to be applied to a surface after identifying the type of dirt and surface, as well as removing dirt.

Detergents

The basic substance used for cleaning is water, which by itself does not work very well. I t tends to form a "skin" round itself a property called *surface tension* which stops it getting deep down into the dirt. Water also does not dissolve fats and oils found as part of To make up for this a group of chemicals are added to the water. The name of this group is a detergent, and is made up like this:

Surfactant: A chemical that is able to reduce surface tension and can combine with both fat and water at the same time. This lets the water get right down to the dirt or penetrate it, breaking it up into small bits emulsifying it, and keeping it broken up, suspending it.

Alkaline

Surfactants on their own do not work very well because acids found in dirt stop them working, so alkaline builders are also added. These neutralise the acids and stop the emulsions breaking down thus stabilising them. Alkaline also react with fats and oils to form soap, a process called saponification, and the soap made helps clean the surface as well.

Water

Because the reaction of hard water with soap forms scum, water softners are added to stop scum being made. These chemicals then made up the basic detergent. To this group can be added a witches brew of chemicals to help out or improve the performance. Among these are nonredeposition agents, which help the surfactant suspend dirt. Foamers which provide the foam, oxidising agents which remove stains, Buffers which control the rate of release of alkaline, and perfumes, Dyes and Preservatives and Thickeners.

Disinfection and Disinfectants

Before any useful progress can be made with developing proper cleaning and disinfect ion techniques in the kitchen, everybody needs to be using the same words to mean the same thing. Disinfection is a process intended to destroy (or remove) micro-organisms, i.e. germs. It does not necessarily have to destroy or remove them all, but just reduce them to a level, which will not harm health or the quality of food. A chemical agent used for disinfection.

Points to remember about disinfection are that the process is a relative one, and that all germs do not necessarily have to be killed or removed. Thus the surface of a floor, which comes nowhere near cooked food, can have a fairly high number of germs on it and not affect health or the quality of food. A work surface however, used for the preparation of cream or cooked meats will have to be almost free of germs before it can be considered safe.

Both surfaces, one with a higher level of germs than the other, can be thought of as disinfected, even though they are not to the same standard, as long as the germs present will not harm health. In the case of a floor, ordinary cleaning with a detergent will often remove sufficient numbers of germs to avoid hard to health, so the process of cleaning can, in this case, be a process of disinfection, even though a disinfectant as such has not been used.

Disinfectants do not have to be strong smelling or highly coloured to work well. The chemical, not the smell, does the work. Disinfectants need to be used on all surfaces and utensils where the cleaning process does not remove sufficient number of germs to avoid danger to health or damage to the quality of food. Generally, the only places in the kitchen where either will be involved is where "sensitive" foods are handled, or for utensils that come into contact with "sensitive" foods, such as:

a) Sandwich preparation areas

b) Gateaux.assembly areas

c) Refrigerators and cold stores where cooked foods are stored.

d) Cooked food set down in the cooking area.

The main thing to remember is that it is usually only food contact surfaces to which disinfection should be applied on a routine basis. The reason for disinfection is to prevent indirect cross contamination. Because germs will survive on even visibly clean surfaces, any surface that has had a raw product placed on it can harbor millions of germs even after cleaning.

If a sensitive food is then placed on that surface, it will then be contaminated by those germs, even though no direct contact has occurred between the two classes of product. The best example of this can be found in the larder type situation, where raw meat may be cut onto a table which is then just cleaned and afterwards used for cold meat salad assembly.

Further indirect contamination can also occur when containers and packages containing raw products come into contact with surfaces, which are later touched by sensitive foods. The use of disinfectants between contacts however will remove the possibility of cross contamination. One important point to remember though is that disinfection has nothing to do with cleaning. The two processes are sometimes carried out at the same time, using a sanitiser but this does not alter the fact that two processes have in fact been carried out.

Kitchen Hazards

The following is a list of the main hazards that may effect the kitchen worker, with brief precautions, for inclusion where relevant, in the unit safety policy:

1. Handling knives and other cutting tools: Always follow knife drill.

2. Operating dangerous machinery: Food slicers, mincers, peelers etc. Always obey specific instructions relating to machinery.
3. Spillages and obstructions on floor: Work clean and wipe up spillages the moment they occur. Keep passages and other traffic areas free from obstruction.
4. Fire: Learn and obey the fire drills.
5. Misuse of mechanical or electrical equipment: Never use equipment for any other purpose than the purpose for which it was intended. Report all faults and do not use defective equipment. Never attempt to put a fault right yourself.
6. Misuse or incorrect storage of cleaning chemicals: Always use chemicals as directed. Always store in the place al located in the original marked containers.
7. Refuse handling and storage: Keep broken glass separate from other refuse in the kitchen. Do not al low refuse to build up in \ the kitchen and cause a fire hazard.
8. Lifting and Carrying: Do not attempt to carry anything that is awkward or heavy, without getting help.
9. Reaching high places: Always use steps or the correct means of access. Do not use chairs, boxes or other articles.
10. Running in the kitchen area: Never run, always walk. Look before you move
11. Stacking goods: Make sure shelving is secure and can take the intended weight.

    Note and obey warnings on packages about stacking heights. Never stack sharp objects where they can fall and cause injury.
12. Gas appliances: Use correctly. Turn off after use. Report all gas leaks the moment they are noticed.

Other hazards may exist, which will be brought to your attention in company memoranda, and where appropriate, in further D.

Safe Use of Chef's Knives and other Dangerous Hand Tools

The dangers of knives are obvious, and under working pressures accidents can happen all too easily, Basic common sense is the key to safety, bearing in mind the following points:

1. Always use the right knife for the job for which it was designed, on the correct cutting surface. Keep your hands and knife handles clean and free from grease as far as possible. Never misuse knives.
2. Make sure that knives are kept in good condition, that handles are kept undamaged and secure. Keep blades in the same good condition and keep them sharp. Never use blunt knives.
3. Never carry knives blade upwards, protect the blade with a sheath or scabbard or carry knives in boxes or trays. Never run while carrying a knife, and for normal movement during jobs, carry the knife blade downwards by your side.
4. Always cut with a knife away from your person. For fine work form a "bridge" with your fingers and cut between the "bridge".
5. Always cut with the work piece firmly placed on a secure surface. Never work with the work piece raised, unless of course you are peeling, with the correct knife. Work in an area where you will be undisturbed and not "bumped" by passing traffic.
6. Never put sharp knives or other sharp tools into sinks full of water and leave them there: when washing knives in a sink, clean them one at a time, keeping

hold of the handle all the time. When cleaning the blade, always wipe downwards from the blunt side

7. Never under any circumstances, hold or handle a sharp knife by the blade.

8. Always store knives in scabbards or the correct container, and always with the blade pointing away from you. Never mix in knives with unprotected blades in with other tools or articles.

Because of the risk of very serious injury while handling sharp knives, even if serious injury is rare, a rubber bandage should always be close to hand where these knives are handled.

Food Poisoning

The nature of food poisoning is generally well understood, even if it is a contradiction in terms. Food sustains life, poison destroy it. However for reference a definition of food poisoning is included here, with explanations:

Food poisoning is an illness brought about in a person by the consumption of food contaminated by noxious materials of micro-organisms. A distinction is made between food poisoning and diseases of a specific nature that are carried by food, such as Typhoid, Brucellosis or Diphtheria. These are known as Food Borne Diseases.

Generally food poisoning is considered to have occurred when it is caused by:

— *Fungi*: Moulds in the substance of the food or harmful fungi mistakenly consumed as edible fungi mushroom etc.

— *Chemicals*: Those less readily known as poison such as lead arsenic or antimony as well as substances like weed killer that has contaminated food.

— *Bacteria*: Certain specific groups of bacteria such as:
   - — Salmonellae
   - — Clostridium perfringens (formerly welchi)
   - — Staphlococci

3

Food Hygiene

Contaminated food represents one of the greatest health risks to a population and is a leading cause of disease outbreaks and transmission. Food that is kept too long can go bad and often contains toxic chemicals or pathogens, and food-stuffs that are eaten raw, such as fruits or vegetables, can become contaminated by dirty hands, unclean water or flies and other such vectors. Improperly prepared food can also cause chemical poisoning. Half cooked or over cooked food for example hard boiled eggs and over cooked meat are bad for health.

To promote good health, therefore, food should be properly stored and prepared.

In many urban centres food is bought and consumed at eating-houses (cafes, restaurants or canteens). If basic health and safety rules for storing, preparing and handling food are not followed in the eating-houses; these places will represent a health hazard for the customers and may cause serious disease outbreaks. The most important aspects of food hygiene in these establishments relate to sanitation, water supply and personal cleanliness:

— Eating-houses should have clean water for washing and drinking, and separate sanitation facilities, away from the kitchen area, for customers, cooks and food-handlers.

— The staff should have clean uniforms each day and have regular medical check-ups.
— The cooks, chefs and waiters should be the most particular in their own personal hygiene so as to prevent any contamination of food handled by them.
— Food to be served should be prepared fresh always and any that is spilled or not used should be disposed off.
— The kitchens and eating areas must be kept clean and free of vermin and insects.
— Eating-houses should also be well-ventilated, with adequate lighting.

Water Sanitation

Water is essential in food preparation. It is used to wash food before cooking, it is used to act as a cooking medium, it is used to clean the containers of food before and after preparation and it is used also as the most important beverage Therefore, it is essential that all water meant for drinking and cooking purposes should be free from pathogenic bacteria.

Water used for making ice must also be potable. The ice may be used to cool foods or added to cold drinks. Thus it is important to ensure that the ice we sometimes buy be made from potable water. Some of the diseases, which can be spread by the use of contaminated water, are cholera, typhoid, paratyphoid, bacillary dysentery and amoebic dysentery.

Water, which is free from pathogenic bacteria and is palatable, is known as potable water. The necessity of a potable water supply in the home and place of work can never be overemphasised. It is also important in institutions preparing, processing and serving food. Apart from the primary precaution to ensure that water be free from harmful bacteria, it is also necessary to make it palatable. For example, water may contain dissolved salts or minerals, which may give it a brackish taste. For specific uses such as chemical analyses water may have to be given special treatment with resins to remove dissolved impurities or salts. We will concern ourselves mainly with the treatment of water to render it safe for potable purposes.

In India, even though the necessity of using 'pure water' has been known for centuries, there was no safe and protected water supply up to 1949 for as much as 81 per cent of the population who stay mostly in the villages. The National Water Supply and Sanitation Programme was launched in 1954 as a part of the Health Plan to assist the States in their urban and rural water supply and sanitation schemes so as to provide adequate water supply and sanitation facilities in the whole country. 1979- 2,108 had provided towns with water benefiting an urban population of one hundred million people.

217 towns with a population of forty million people (about 36 per cent of the urban population) had been covered by partial sewerage system. Of the 5,76,000 villages it is estimated that more than two lakh problem villages remained to be covered with potable water supply as on April 1, 1980. Efforts are being made to meet the water and sanitation needs of the entire country. Even today the average Indian, educated or uneducated, a villager or a city-dweller, is very particular about seeing that the vessels used for storage of water is not contaminated in the home. So it is not the use in the home but the source of the water supply, which may be suspect.

Water Contamination Sources

The usual source of contamination of water is through the seepage of sewage. Sewage can be a carrier of many pathogenic bacteria because many healthy persons may be 'carriers' of pathogenic bacteria without being affected themselves. Persons who are suffering from enteric diseases will also contribute to the presence of bacteria in sewage. The disposal of sewage is not paid much attention to, especially in the rural communities, where a human excreta is deposited near shallow wells, ponds or even rivers; contamination from this source is widespread.

In cities, the huge influx of population, which results in rapid formation of hutment dwellings without proper sanitary and water facilities, develop into a health hazard. Sufficient water is not available usually at such dwellings and the use of water from any source is resorted to, sometimes even gutter water being used. It is not that the hutment dwellers are not aware of the hazards involved, but they have no other alternative. There is no facility for drainage and the used water and sewage stand, encouraging breeding of mosquitoes and flies. These pests carry and spread pathogens from sewage to nearby localities, thus creating health problems. Exposed ready-to-eat foods sold in such localities may be contaminated by the flies.

Another difficulty experienced in cities with protected water supplies is the difficulty of maintaining a positive pressure in all pipelines. In cities many of the pipelines have become very old and unless there is a continuous flow of water into them with a positive pressure there is a possibility of seepage of bacteria, from sewage into water pipes. With limited supply of water available, in many Indian cities, all the pipes can never be holding water all the 24 hours. This is a problem, which does cause concern. The effluents from many industries, which are at present mostly discharged into rivers, are another source of contamination; this problem is assuming serious proportions.

Many of these effluents use up much of the oxygen from the water with the result that fish and other aquatic animals are unable to survive. Foul smell emanates from such streams, due to anaerobic decomposition (putrefaction) of dead fish, thus making the water unfit for human consumption.

Water Treatment

It is thus essential that water used for potable purposes be free from pathogenic bacteria. The best precaution one can take is to prevent the source of water from contamination with sewage. In villages this can be done by constructing cement sides to deep wells to prevent bacteria from seeping through the soil and gaining entrance in the water. Well water, which may be contaminated, can be purified by the addition of bleaching powder. Bleaching powder on reaction with water releases chlorine, which is capable of killing pathogenic organisms.

In villages where there is no treated water, drinking water should preferably be boiled and then cooled. This would destroy all the pathogenic bacteria. Water used for cooking need not be boiled, as it would be boiled anyway during cooking. Water used for washing, cleaning need not be boiled as long as it is not foul smelling and does not contain any suspended impurities. In cities and towns where it is necessary to supply a large population with water, effective methods have to be used for the purification of water. The source of water is usually a lake in which the water is allowed to stand. This results in most of the suspended impurities settling down. Further the action of sunlight and the paucity of food results in the destruction of bacteria.

In the next stage, which may consist of a filtration through sand most of the bacteria are eliminated. As an added precaution water supplies to cities are chlorinated.

This may either be done by the addition of bleaching powder, or as is done in most of the cities, by the injection of liquid chlorine. To make sure that the bacteria, which may have entered into the pipelines through seepage when there is no positive pressure, additional chlorination is resorted to at different locations during the transportation of water from the lake to city reservoirs. This is understandable when it is realised that the source of water may be 60 to 70 km away from the city. Water may be rendered potable by use of water filter in the home.

Pesticide residue can pose a serious problem in the diet. There are certain precautions, which you can take to reduce dietary exposure to this hazard. These are:

— Thoroughly rinse and scrub fruits and vegetables. Peel them if appropriate.

— Remove outer leaves of leafy vegetables, such as cabbage and lettuce.

— Trim fat from meat, poultry and fish; discard oils and fats in broths and drippings.

— Throw back the big fish-the little ones have less time to take up and concentrate pesticides and other harmful residues.

All vegetables and fruits either from bazar or grown in one's own farm would have to be cleaned, and prepared for either eating directly or cooking. The dirt or dust, which we find on foods as we buy them, can be carrier of spores of microorganisms. Therefore, all exposed food must be washed with clean water before use. Outer layers, skins of plant material contain thousands of microorganisms and must be washed thoroughly before use. If any parts of fruits and vegetables are bruised these should be trimmed to reduce contamination. The skin, hair, feathers, intestines of animals harbour a number of microorganisms. It is, therefore, necessary to remove these, before animal products are prepared for human consumption.

Food comes into contact with human hands during harvesting, storage, preparation and service. It is important that food handlers be free from any communicable diseases-colds, any other respiratory ailment, cuts or boils, as they may be responsible for transferring these to the food thereby spreading the infection to persons consuming the food. Human hair, nasal discharge, skin can also be source of microorganisms. Therefore, persons handling food, must wash hands with soap before starting preparation, and refrain from touching hair or wiping nose during food preparation.

Food sanitation is a way of life. It can never be overemphasised. A number of gastrointestinal disorders, such as diarrhea, cholera and communicable diseases such as typhoid, septic sore throat, diphtheria, dysentery, etc., are communicated by use of contaminated water or food. Therefore, it is very important that sanitary handling of food and water is religiously adhered to.

Food Contamination

Food may be contaminated if the:

— Water used for washing or cleaning is not potable.

— Soil adhering to foods grown close to ground is not completely removed.

— Containers or utensils used for storage and preparation are not clean.

— Personnel handling food have unhygienic habits.

— Personnel handling food suffer from communicable diseases.

Equipment Sanitation

It is necessary that all equipment coming in contact with food be kept clean. This includes knives, meat mincers, blenders, rolling pins, wooden boards, metal and porcelain dishes, utensils, etc. They should be scrubbed, cleaned with detergent and water and then rinsed with potable water. It is a good practice to see that such equipment are dipped in hot water at 80°C for at least 30 seconds or more and then allowed to drain dry. This sanitary step is especially important during epidemics such as infective hepatitis (infective jaundice), cholera, etc. Parts of blenders, mixers, etc., should be inspected after cleaning to ensure that there is no food material left over. If allowed to remain they could allow harmful microorganisms to grow and spoil the food.

Equipment made of plastic and other such material which cannot withstand high temperatures need not be given the dip in hot water but should be given the other treatments and then allowed to drain dry. In villages it is a common practice to scrub utensils and dishes with ash and then rinse them with water. The utensils and dishes are then allowed to dry in the sun. The alkaline ash acts as a good agent for killing any microorganisms adhering to the utensils and a sanitary effect is produced by drying in the sun both because of heat and the ultraviolet rays.

Insects and Rodents Control

One of the common insects contaminating foods is the housefly. These have minute hair on their legs and thus can be the carriers of harmful bacteria depending on where they come from. It is possible that they may carry faecal matter or other such sources of pathogenic bacteria and deposit it on the food. Another insect, which can also be a source of contamination in the same way as the housefly, is, the cockroach. These insects, which usually prefer darkness, have been known to cause diarrhea and dysentery.

Apart from these two common ones, there are innumerable insects ranging from the larvae found in wheat and rice to locusts, which can cause serious damage to food. Rodents, which include rats, mice and bandicoots, not only consume large quantities of food, thus contributing to the overall shortage of food in the country, but may also be the carriers of diseases such as plague. The presence of insects, insect fragments, rodent excreta and other matter of insect and rodent origin (even though it may not necessarily be dangerous to health) is aesthetically resented by consumers.

Health authorities condemn such food as unfit for consumption because it indicates poor practices of sanitation where the food was prepared. It is thus essential that preventive measures be taken to exclude the entry of insects and rodents in the house, especially in the cooking and serving areas. This can be done by:

— Keeping the prepared food in cupboards with wire-netting,

— Filling cracks, fissures in the walls and flooring which are usually the places where insects breed and multiply.

— Covering drains, holes, etc., with wire gauze so as to prevent the entry of rodents.

Precautions such as these if taken in villages and small towns where people normally stay in independent homes would certainly prevent the entry of insects and rodents. In large cities, however, where each building may have many apartments, unless measures are taken by the whole community, there is always a danger of insects and rodents travelling from one apartment to another. The control of insects and rodents can be carried oat in several ways of which the most common one practised in the home is spraying or dusting with an insecticide. Fumigation may be resolved to in large godowns, factories, etc., as it destroys insects and rodents.

Sprays or dustings make use of chlorinated hydrocarbons (such as DDT, TDE, aldrin, dieldrin, etc.) and the organic phosphorus compounds (such as Parathion, Malathion, Systrex, etc.) as the active ingredient for killing the insect. Baits in which chemicals may be mixed with food are also successful in getting rid of pests. Examples of these are "Tygon" in which a chemical is mixed with sugar and a home-made mixture of boric powder and bengalgram dal flour, which when ingested by cockroaches results in their death.

Warfrain may be mixed with food and used as a bait for the elimination of rodents. It must be noted that insecticides are poisonous, and must be used in very small amounts only where needed. If used indiscriminately these are likely to enter our bodies and harm us after a period of time. It is important to store these out of reach of children and away from food, to prevent accidents.

Good Sanitation Rules

— Tie hair neatly before starting food preparation. Use hair net or cap if necessary. Wash hands thoroughly with soap and water before starting preparation.

— Wash fruits, vegetables, cereals and beans thoroughly before preparation with potable water. Boil milk in a clean container as soon as possible after receipt and keep covered. Bottles of milk need to be rinsed thoroughly with water and then washed with soap and water.

— Use potable water in food preparation.

— Boil water used for drinking for preparation of cold beverages, if the purity of water is not guaranteed.

— Utensils and equipment used for preparation. Should be scrupulously cleaned.

— Cooked food should be stored covered, preferably in the container in which it is cooked.

— Left over foods such as rice, vegetables should be stored either in a refrigerator kept in a pan of cold water. Reheating before use is advisable.

Food Sanitation Programmes

Food Sanitation is protection from contamination. With this in mind, all functions and operations must be included in a sanitation programme. All food products must be protected from contamination from receiving through distribution. Sanitation is a dynamic and ongoing function and cannot be sporadic or something that can be turned on once a day, once a week, etc. Therefore, another definition could be: "sanitation is a way of life".

Temperature Control

The primary rule of sanitation is to pay strict attention to food temperatures.

— Avoid prolonged holding in the danger zone.

— Provide functional thermometers to all food storage boxes.

— Monitor the temperature on serving lines on a regular frequency.

— Thaw frozen foods under refrigeration or under cold water.

— Do not thaw foods at room temperature.

Hygiene and Personnel Practices

Regardless of type of processing or food handling

operation, the number one consideration in food sanitation is people. It is people who set the rules, follow the rules, and also break the rules of sanitation. A sanitation programme is as good as the attitude, willingness, and efforts of people. That is why the most important aspect of a sanitation programme is ongoing personnel training. It is essential that the full meaning of sanitation and its wide economic scope be accepted by everyone concerned in the food system-including management. Personnel training should include appropriate sanitation principles and food handling practices, manufacturing controls, and personal hygiene practices.

Sanitation Principles and Food Handling Practices

Personnel training should instill and nurture an understanding of the processing steps and technologies for each product manufactured or handled and where potential problems exist, and create a keen desire to satisfy and guard the consumers' interests.

Production personnel must be trained in the critical elements of the operations for which they are responsible, in the importance of these operations, monitoring these operations, and in action to be taken when these operations are not controlled. Certain industries have developed certification programmes for operators of essential heat-processing equipment. If such programmes don't exist for a given processing segment, it is important that specific training programmes be developed for such personnel.

Hygienic Practices

Communicable diseases/Injuries

Persons known to be suffering from, or known to be carriers of a disease likely to be transmitted through food, must be restricted from any food-handling area. Likewise, persons afflicted with infected wounds, skin infections, sores, etc., must also be restricted from these areas. Any persons with open cuts or wounds should not handle food unless the injury is completely protected by a secure, waterproof covering.

Hand-washing

Facilities with hot water for hand-washing must be provided and must be convenient to food handling areas. All personnel involved in food handling must thoroughly wash hands with soap under warm-running, potable water. Hands must also be washed after handling contaminated materials and after using toilet facilities. Where required, employees must use disinfectant hand dips.

Personal cleanliness and conduct

— Personal cleanliness must be maintained while involved in food handling operations:

— Sanitary protective clothing, hair covering, and footwear must be worn and maintained in a clean, sanitary manner.

— Gloves, if worn, must be clean and sanitary.

— All food-handling personnel must remove objects from their person which may fall into or contaminate the food product.

— Tobacco, gum, and food are not permitted in food-handling areas.

Personnel and visitor access to specific food-product handling areas must be restricted. Personnel involved in raw product handling must not be allowed in processing or finished product areas. Foot baths and hand dips, where required, must be properly maintained and used. Color coding of clothing, maintenance and other equipment should be used to clearly identify raw vs. processed product operations.

Surroundings

Outside surroundings

Outside surroundings should be evaluated for sources of contamination such as vermin, bird harborage areas, drainage problems, odor problems, debris, refuse, and pollution-smoke, dust, other contaminants. Appropriate steps must be taken to contain and control any potential sources of contamination.

Buildings and facilities

The two most important overall elements of any food-processing and -handling facility is that it should be cleanable, and so designed and constructed that it prevents entrance or harborage of pests or other sources of contamination. Unfortunately, many existing facilities do not readily meet these essential elements.

The facility should have floors, walls, and ceilings constructed of suitable, approved materials which are durable, smooth, impervious and easily cleaned. Walls should be light colored and well-joined, and floors should be adequately sloped for drainage to trapped outlets. Openings to outside and/or non-food-processing or -handling rooms or facilities must be sealed. Instrument panels should be appropriately locked and sealed to prevent harborage of insects. Windows and doors must be tight and close-fitting. And doors in food-processing areas self-closing.

Overhead structures should be situated and constructed to prevent contamination of the food products, and lighting is to be adequate with properly sealed, safety type overhead fixtures.

Heating, Ventilation, and Air Conditioning (HVAC)

Systems must be designed and installed to prevent build-up of heat, steam, condensation, or dust, and to remove contaminated air. Positive air pressure is required in microbiologically sensitive areas. HVAC systems should be designed to be cleanable, and air intakes located to prevent intake of contaminated air. Appropriate traps and vents are to be used throughout. There should be no potential of cross connections existing between human waste effluent and other wastes in the plant. Appropriate vacuum breakers or air breaks must be used.

Waste facilities

Facilities designed to prevent contamination should provide for the sanitary storage of waste and inedible material prior to their removal from plant or surroundings. Waste containers are to be clearly identified.

In general, the facilities and various non-product contact surfaces and equipment must be evaluated to assess potential for food-product contamination. Shielding from overhead contamination should be provided as deemed necessary. Examples include: shielding over food product fillers or bottle conveyers, shielding from refrigeration unit drip in coolers, sneeze guards on food service serving lines, etc.

A well-designed food-processing or -handling facility is constructed to minimise traffic to prevent contamination. It is desirable to have a product flow-through that physically and operationally separates raw product functions from processing functions and finished product functions in order to avoid cross-contamination. Boiler and engineering rooms must always be separated from food-processing and -handling areas.

Sanitary facilities

Self-closing doors must be provided for all washroom facilities. Washrooms, lunchrooms, and change rooms must be separate from-and not directly entered from-food-processing and -handling areas. Such facilities are to be properly ventilated and maintained.

Sufficient numbers of handwashing sinks, with hot and cold potable water, soap, sanitary hand drying supplies or devices, must be provided in washrooms. A sufficiency of suitably located handwashing sinks are also necessary in food processing and handling areas. Hand-washing sinks should be separate from sinks used for equipment cleaning and other operations.

A potable water, steam, and ice supply is imperative for sanitary food-processing and handling. Compliance with appropriate regulations and standards must be verified through testing programmes. Water treatments, if applied, must be maintained. Adequate water temperatures and pressures are to be provided in processing areas.

All elements and operations involved with receiving and storage of ingredients, packaging material, and other incoming materials must be evaluated and monitored to prevent potential contamination of the food product manufactured. Incoming materials must be received into an area which is separated from processing areas. Only safe, approved food-grade direct and indirect additives andingredients shall be used. Packaging materials used must be safe and approved.

Storage

Where appropriate and applicable, the temperature and

humidity of storage rooms for raw materials, ingredients, packaging materials, and food should be maintained and monitored.

Foods returned from retail outlets must be clearly identified and stored in a designated area for appropriate disposition. Storage conditions need be such that the safety of the returned food is not compromised.

Detergents, sanitisers, or other chemicals must be properly labeled, stored and used in a manner to prevent contamination of food, packaging materials, and food contact surfaces. Chemicals must be stored in a dry, well-ventilated area which is separate from food handling areas.

All food-processing and -handling rooms and other rooms must be maintained in a clean, sanitary manner. A major source of plant contamination is from custodial personnel and equipment. All custodial brushes and equipment must be in good repair as well as being clean and sanitary.

The overall requirement for design of equipment for food-processing and -handling operations is that it be cleanable and maintained in such a manner as to prevent contamination. Food-contact surface equipment standards-of varying thoroughness-have been developed for segments of the food industry.

Equipment Installation

It does little good to have equipment which is designed to be cleanable, but which is installed in such a manner or location as to preclude its cleanability. Adequate space must be provided within and around equipment, and equipment must be accessible for cleaning, sanitising, maintenance, and inspection.

A sanitary operations facility has a preventive maintenance programme which monitors equipment maintenance procedures. Such a programme specifies necessary servicing intervals, replacement parts, etc. Protocols and calibration methods must be established for all equipment that could impact on food safety. These include:

— thermometers,

— pH meters,

— water activity meters,

— refrigeration controls,

— scales,

— recording thermometers,

— hygrometers, and other equipment.

All reagents used for monitoring and verification must be documented and stored properly. Appropriate monitors must be used.

Thoroughly evaluate the effectiveness of cleaning and sanitising programmes. Consult a reputable cleaning and sanitising supplier and follow recommendedprocedures for cleaning and sanitising both food- product contact and non-product contact surfaces in specific operations.

An adequate pest control programme is necessary for sanitary operation of a food-processing or -handling facility. Effectiveness of the pest-control programme should be verified on a regular frequency. An important part of food sanitation programme is having a working product-recall system in place. The recall programme establishes procedures to be implemented in the event of a product recall. Written recall procedures should be established and tested for validity.

Food Poisoning

The nature of food poisoning is generally well understood,

even if it is a contradiction in terms. Food sustains life, poison destroy it A distinction is made between food poisoning and diseases of a specific nature that are carried by food, such as Typhoid, Brucellosis or Diphtheria. These are known as Food Borne Diseases.

Generally food poisoning is considered to have occurred when it is caused by:

— *Fungi*: Moulds in the substance of the food or harmful fungi mistakenly consumed as edible fungi mushroom etc.

— *Chemicals*: Those less readily known as poison such as lead arsenic or antimony as well as substances like weed killer that has contaminated food.

— *Bacteria*: Certain specific groups of bacteria such as Salmonellae, Clostridium perfringens (formerly Welchi), Staphlococci as well as other less well known groups.

— *Viruses*: Certain ill defined and poorly understood viruses known collectively as entero viruses. In some cases, other types of micro-organism may be responsible for food poisoning. As may certain parasites.

Food Poisoning Germs

Germs do not come out of nowhere, nor do they exist everywhere. In a sense, they are parasites that live in or on warm-blooded animals. For that reason, food poisoning germs are very rarely found on fresh fish, and any germs found in your kitchen are at the end of a journey that started with an animal, the source.

To get from that place to the kitchen, germs have to be carried. By themselves they cannot travel very far, inches at the most, and it is rare for them to be carried in the air. The main place to look for the "carrier" is meat, since meat is an animal product, and it is no exaggeration to say that most food poisoning germs, Salmonella certainly, start on the farm and come to the kitchen via the slaughterhouse, meat plants and butchers.

Soil is also a source of food poisoning germs, but only because fields are occupied by animals. Germs that infect fruit and vegetables, or the soil sticking to them still started off their journey with animals, these products are just the carriers. In the same way, cereals and other foods that are known sometimes to be infected with food poisoning germs are only a passing home in the life of a germ.

Biologically speaking, human beings are animals so all people who come into contact with food are potential sources. Some types of germs are so common that they are present in the skin of nearly everybody; others are less common, living in the gut. Pests, both rodents and insects, can also be considered as animals, and these are the third major source of germs, so well established that the most common type of Salmonella is named after the mouse. Pests may also carry food poisoning germs from one place to another, from the dustbins to the kitchen for instance, and in this respect they are not the direct source, but carriers, sometimes called "vectors".

For practical purposes in catering, it is not necessary to distinguish between the main source and the carrier. Knowledge of the main sources helps in the understanding of food poisoning control, but to all intents and purposes, everything in the kitchen must be thought of" as a potential source of food poisoning, unless and until active measures have been taken to remove or control that source.

Animal prodicts however will be the main target, since these are the main sources, heat processing, as in milk pasteurization, and cooking being the main line of defence. Cooking is in fact the main barrier between food poisoning and the consumer, and every other activity is supplementary to that.

Carriers

Throughout the history of food borne disease, the carrier has always held a prominent position in the spread of food poisoning. A carrier is an infected person (or animal) that harbours a specific infectious agent without showing any symptoms and acts as a potential source of infection to man. A carrier does not have to have an infection to become infective: Exposure to certain types of bacteria under certain conditions, for instance Salmonella while handling raw meat over a long period, can result in a carrier state.

Carriers therefore are subdivided into groups according to the nature of the state and, sometimes the way they acquired infection, as follows:

— *Healthy* a carrier who has acquired that state without having had any apparent illness.

— *Convalescent* a carrier who has acquired that state as a result of illness associated with the infectious agent carried.

— *Temporary* a carrier who is in the carrier state for a short period of time.

— *Chronic* a carrier who remains infectious for a long period of time.

— *Intermittent* a carrier who excretes infectious material on an irregular basis.

Generally, carriers are dangerous because they excrete infectious material in their faces, which can, by poor personal hygiene or disinfections be transferred to food. The most dangerous type of carrier is the healthy carrier who may remain unrecognized and continue working with food, more so if he/she is intermittent, when even if the carrier state is suspected it may be difficult to detect.

Carriers are detected by stool (faecal) sampling, either after a food poisoning outbreak or on a routine basis. This is an unreliable way, owing to the presence of intermittent carriers. It is estimated that up to 6% of the population are carriers of one sort or another.

Knowledge of what germs need to survive, and what kills them, helps the understanding of how they can be control led in the kitchen. Listed here are some of the main factors:

1. *Food*: The presence or absence of suitable food will affect the survival of most germs. Some germs however will live for years without any recognisable source of food, and others in a state similar to hibernation, called the spore state, can live for centuries.
2 *Type of Food*: Whether the food is liquid or solid, if it is high in sugar or salt content, or if it is either acid or alkaline has a direct bearing on germ survival. "Generally germs prefer a liquid food high in protein content. Sugars and salt above a certain level, high acid levels and to a lesser extent high alkaline foods will tend to destroy germs.
3. *Moisture:* All germs need water to function actively, although spores will survive without it. Even a thin film of condensation will allow active germs to survive.
4 *Heat:* Within a certain range of temperature, roughly between l0°C and 62°C, germs will reproduce. At 37°e the temperature is ideal. Levels above 620e will generally kill germs and levels below 100°C will stop them reproducing.

5. *Time*: Germs need time to reproduce, and they take time to be killed. Heat alone will not kill germs; it is always the combination of temperature at a "certain level for a given time that kills them.
6. *Rate of Heat Application*: Heating to a given temperature very slowly will allow more germs to survive than if that temperature is reached quickly. Fast heat application or sudden changes in temperatures can kill germs even if normally lethal levels are not reached. This is called "heat shock".
7. *Presence of Oxygen*: Some germs need oxygen. These are called aerobes. Others flourish without it and are known as anaerobes. Oxygen is normally present in foods except those that have a high liquid content and have been heavily boiled.
8. *Competition*: The law of the jungle applies even under the microscope and where there are many different bacteria present on a surface they will compete for the same food etc. The weaker ones will die and these are usually the food poisoning germs as these are out of their best environment.
9. *Changing Environment:* Transfer of germs suddenly from one type of surface to another can kill them, even though they could have lived on either. So many factors affect survival that it is perhaps a surprise that they live at all.

Prevention of Food Poisoning

With a very wide variety of factors influencing the survival of food poisoning bacteria, (germs) it is difficult to always bear everything in mind. Many of the factors in any case are outside the control of the caterer. The nature of the food you work with, its moisture content and to an extent, rates of heat application are all governed by menu requirements. Food poisoning in catering however can be successfully prevented by controlling three factors: Contamination, Temperature, and Time.

— *Contamination*: involved the preparation of clean food, for it is in "dirt" that germs survive, adequate cooking procedures to destroy germs that escape the net, the prevention of cross contamination between cooked and raw foods, not allowing people or pests to contaminate and destroying any contamination in the kitchen by disinfections.

— *Temperature*: involves not giving bacteria the temperatures they like for reproduction. Keeping food either hot (above 63°C) or cold (below 10°C) whenever possible.

— *Time*: Since bacteria need time as well as temperature to reproduce, this involves not giving them enough time, when temperatures are such that germs will be able to reproduce. In normal kitchen practice it is not possible to make sure that food is completely uncontaminated, nor would it be a good thing to have sterile food. Thus as long as only a small amount of contamination (and with it food poisoning bacteria) is present no harm would be done.

This failure to remove contamination will only be dangerous if germs are allowed to multiply in number and to do this they need the right temperature. It is not always possible to avoid these temperature conditions so you fail again on this factor, so where this happens, by limiting the time available for germs to multiply, safety can still be achieved. This is the "Fail -Safe" approach. You try, but fail, to control contamination and likewise with temperature and time, but by controlling each factor in relation to the other, when you do fail, you fail safe.

Sensitive Foods

All foods can cause food poisoning but some are known

to cause disease more often than others, owing to their nature, which particularly encourages the growth of bacteria. Sensitive foods are foods, which, by their nature will provide favorable conditions for the growth of bacteria and are prepared or sold in such a way that tends to, allow their survival and multiplication. Examples of these foods, in the catering operation, are as follows:

— Any cooked meat, especially poultry, whether served hot or cold.
— Cooked meat products, whether served hot or cold.
— Milk, cream and artificial cream, and dairy products (Except cheese, butter etc.)
— Eggs and egg products, other than those usec baking.
— Shellfish, prawns and similar sea foods.
— Less commonly dessicated coconut, rice and corn flour.

As a general rule, any product that is protein based, and is either served uncooked, or after it has been cooked or processed, is a sensitive food. Understanding what sensitive foods are is one of the most important steps in preventing food poisoning, as most of your energy devoted to prevention should be concentrated on these foods.

Temperatures, Foods and Germs

The Control of temperature is one of the keys to preventing food poisoning: Unfortunately there are many different temperatures to remember and, with the increasing use of Centigrade units remembering is difficult. Reproduced here are 50me of the important temperatures:

100°C Boiling Point of Water. Most but not all germs are killed in seconds; some though survive up to 3 hours.

80°C Minimum temperature for baine marie water.

72°C	Minimum temperature for the centre of cooked meats intended for cooling and storage. * 63°C Upper limit for germ growth. Minimum temperature for the centre of cooked meat.
37°C	Temperature at which food poisoning grows best. (Blood heat).
22°C	Typical Kitchen Temperature.
10°C	Lower limit of germ growth. Maximum temperature for the storage of all perishable foods.
0°C	Freezing point of water. Ideal temperature for raw meat storage.
5°C	Ideal temperature for fish storage.
18°C	Frozen food storage: deep freezers.

The critical range, as far as food poisoning is concerned, is between l0o C and 63°C, called the danger zone. Within this range germs will reproduce, and the closer they come to 37°C the faster they grow, doubling in number at a peak of every 15 minutes for some types.

Cross Contamination

Stopping contamination is one of the most important things that must be done if food poisoning is to be prevented. Cross is the process of passing on germs (contamination) from uncooked, or unprocessed foods, to those foods which have been cooked or processed. For general purposes it is always assumed that cooked and processed foods are free from germs and that uncooked foods are always contaminated.

Hygiene during Food Processing

Food processing is the set of methods and techniques used

to transform raw ingredients into food for consumption by humans. Food processing often takes clean, harvested or slaughtered and butchered components and uses these to produce attractive and marketable food products. Similar process are used to produce animal feed. Following are common food processing techniques:

- Removal of unwanted outer layers, such as potato peeling or the skinning of Peaches
- Chopping or slicing, of which examples include potato chips, diced carrot, or candied peel.
- Mincing and macerating
- Liquefaction, such as to produce fruit juice
- Emulsification
- Cooking, such as boiling, broiling, frying, steaming or grilling
- Mixing
- Addition of gas such as air entrainment for bread or gasification of soft drinks
- Proofing
- spray drying

Food processing dates back to the prehistoric ages when crude processing incorporated slaughtering, various types of cooking, such as over fires, smoking, steaming, oven baking), fermenting, sun drying and preserving with salt. Foods preserved this way were a common part of warriors and sailor's diets up until the introduction of canned food. These crude processing techniques remained essentially the same until the advent of the industrial revolution. Modern food processing technology in the 19th and 20th century were largely developed to serve military needs.

Nicolas Appert developed a vacuum bottling process to supply troops in the French army with food, which would eventually lead to tinning and then canning by

Peter Durand in 1810. Although initially expensive and somewhat hazardous due to lead used in the cans, canned goods would later become a staple around the world. Pasteurization, discovered by Louis Pasteur in 1862 was a significant advance in ensuring micro-biological safety of food..

In the 20th century, World War II, the space race and the developing consumer society in the developed world furthered the development of food processing with advances such as spray drying, juice concentrates, freeze drying and the introduction of artificial sweetners, colorants, and preservatives such as sodium benzoate and saccharine. In the late 20th century products such as dried instant soups, reconstituted fruits and juices, and self cooking meals such as MRE food ration were developed.

Benefits of food processing includes toxin removal, preservation, improving flavour, easing marketing and distribution tasks, and increasing food consistency. In addition, it increases seasonal availability of many foods, enables transportation of delicate perishable foods across long distances, and makes many kinds of foodstuffs safe to eat by removing the microorganisms.

Modern supermarkets would not be feasible without modern food processing techniques, long voyages would not be possible, and military campaigns would be significantly more difficult and costly to execute. Modern food processing also improves the quality of life for allergics, diabetics, and other people who cannot consume some common food elements. Food processing can also add extra nutrients.

Food processing can lower the nutritional value of some foods. Some preservatives added or created during processing such as nitrites or sulphites may cause adverse health effects on some consumers. In addition, high quality and hygiene standards must be maintained to ensure consumer safety and failures to maintain adequate standards can have serious health consequences. In general, fresh food that has not been processed other than by washing and simple kitchen preparation, may be expected to contain a higher propotion of naturally occuring vitamins, fibre and minerals than the equivalent product processed by the food industry. However fresh matereials are more liable to early spoilage and are often unsuited to long distance transportion from source to shelf.

Sanitation of Equipment

It is necessary that all equipment coming in contact with food be kept clean. This includes knives, meat mincers, blenders, rolling pins, wooden boards, metal and porcelain dishes, utensils, etc. They should be scrubbed, cleaned with detergent and water and then rinsed with potable water. It is a good practice to see that such equipment are dipped in hot water at 80°C for at least 30 seconds or more and then allowed to drain dry. This sanitary step is especially important during epidemics such as infective hepatitis, cholera, etc.

Parts of blenders, mixers, etc., should be inspected after cleaning to ensure that there is no food material left over. If allowed to remain they could allow harmful microorganisms to grow and spoil the food. Equipment made of plastic and other such material which cannot withstand high temperatures need not be given the dip in hot water but should be given the other treatments and then allowed to drain dry.

In villages it is a common practice to scrub utensils and dishes with ash and then rinse them with water. The utensils and dishes are then allowed to dry in the sun. The alkaline ash acts as a good agent for killing any microorganisms adhering to the utensils and a sanitary effect is produced by drying in the sun both because of heat and the ultraviolet rays.

Food Processors

Modern food processors come in three basic sizes: full, compact, and mini. No matter what size they are, however, the basic components are the same: a motor, a bowl with a lid and feed tube, and a set of attachments. The motor is housed in the base of the appliance, and it is the heaviest part of the device. Full-size machines generally have larger, more powerful motors, and can weigh more than 20 lbs (9 kg). This weight has a utilitarian value: The heaviness of the base gives the appliance stability and ensures that it doesn't move around while the motor is running.

Though the first food processor bases were clad only in white, hard plastic, today they are available in a range of stylish colours and with metal and plastic finishes, ensuring that your appliance will fit in with your kitchen decor. From the motor, a shaft extends upward to power the attachments. The bowl, which is usually made of durable, transparent plastic, fits onto this shaft and locks into position. The lid, usually made of the same material, locks onto the top of the bowl; in many older models, engaging the locking mechanism turns on the motor, but newer models generally have an on/off switch or button.

The lid has a feed tube fitted with a plunger. You can insert food into the device through this feed tube, pushing it down with the plunger. Some models have wider and narrower feed tubes for use with larger and smaller food items. The size of the bowl varies according to the size of the machine:

— Full-size bowls generally have a capacity of 9 to 13 cups.

— Compact-size bowls can accommodate 5 to 7 cups.

— Mini-size bowls can fit 2 to 5 cups.

Some models come with large and small bowls for use with the same base. The attachments fit over the shaft inside the bowl. Standard attachments for a food processor are an S-shaped blade — also known as a sabatier blade — and shredding and slicing discs. The sabatier blade sits at the bottom of the bowl. It consists of two small, curved blades arranged on opposite sides of a central plastic pillar that fits onto the shaft inside the bowl. The blades of the sabatier are usually made of metal, but are sometimes made of hard plastic. You may find that metal blades are preferable because they retain their sharpness longer.

The shredding and slicing discs are made of metal and sit at the top of the bowl, over the shaft. You push food down the feed tube and it contacts the disc, at which point it is grated or sliced into the bowl. The holes on the shredding and slicing discs may yield fine, medium, or coarse bits of food. You can purchase these different versions of the discs separately if they are not included with your food processor. In addition to the standard attachments that came with your food processor, you can supplement your equipment and make your appliance more versatile by buying additional attachments.

Using food processor

The shredding disc quickly and efficiently grates common ingredients like cheese and carrots, and the slicing disc yields perfectly even slices of potatoes and apples in no time at all. You just push the food through the feed tube using the plunger. Chopping, grinding and pureeing involve a little more technique. Let's illustrate this by learning how to make fresh salsa using your processor. You know that fresh salsa contains vegetables such as tomatoes and hot chillies; it can also incorporate ingredients like scallions, garlic, and fresh coriander.

You might be tempted to just throw all your ingredients into the food processor and turn it on, but you'll end up with something more like gazpacho soup than salsa. It's better to work in stages, because the different ingredients in your salsa will have different textures: You want the chillies and garlic pureed so that their flavour is distributed evenly throughout; you want the scallions and coriander finely chopped but not pureed, so that small green pieces are visible; and you want your tomatoes in bite-sized chunks. To achieve this variation in size and texture, you're going to have to introduce the ingredients one or two at a time, processing them in turn.

Since the garlic and chilli need the most processing, let's start with them. Peel a clove of garlic, remove the stem from a hot chilli, and throw them in the bottom of your food processor bowl. Then turn it on. You'll see that the garlic and chilli quickly get chopped up, but if your bowl is large, you might find that they get thrown against the side, away from the blades. You will have to turn off the motor and scrape down the bowl, putting the food pieces nearer to the blades again. You will also find that adding a bit of liquid (a tablespoon of fresh lime juice, water or olive oil would be perfect for your salsa) will help ensure that food thrown against the side of the bowl drips back down to the bottom rather quickly.

Pulsing is one of the most important food-processor techniques; it allows you to keep an eye on the texture of your food to ensure that you don't over-process it. After 10 to 15 one-second pulses, and several scrape-downs, your garlic and chilli should be pureed. Now let's add the scallion and coriander. Be sure that you wash all the vegetables well, and trim off the roots and ragged bits.

Mixers

A mixer is a kitchen appliance intended for mixing, folding, beating, and whipping food ingredients. Mixers come in two major variations, hand mixers and stand mixers. A hand mixer, as the name implies, is a hand-held device. It typically consists of a handle mounted over a large enclosure containing the motor, which drives two beaters. The beaters are immersed in the food to be mixed. Hand mixers are often battery-powered.

A stand mixer is essentially the same as a hand mixer, but is mounted on a stand which bears the weight of the device. Stand mixers are larger and have more powerful motors than their hand-held counterparts. They generally have a special bowl that is locked in place while the mixer is operating. Heavy duty commercial models can have bowl capacities in excess of 100 quarts (95 L), but more typical home and commercial models are equipped with bowls of around 4 quarts (4 L).

A typical home stand mixer will include a wire whip for whipping creams and egg whites; a flat beater for mixing batters; and a dough hook for kneading. Mixers should not be confused with blenders. Blenders contain sharp blades and typically operate at higher speeds that chop, liquify, or otherwise break down larger food items. A mixer is a much slower device without blades.

Blenders

A blender is a kitchen appliance used to blend ingredients or puree food. The term typically refers to a stationary, upright electrical device, which is to be distinguished from a hand-powered or electric mixer that may be used for similar purposes. A typical blender is built around a vessel for the ingredients to be blended. At the top of the vessel is a cap to prevent ingredients from escaping when the blender is switched on. At the bottom is a blade assembly, typically removable for cleaning purposes. The bottom seal is most likely watertight. The vessel rests upon a base containing a motor (for turning the blade assembly) with controls on its surface.

Most modern blenders offer a number of possible speeds. In 1922, Stephen Poplawski invented the blender. Stephen Poplawski was the first to put a spinning blade at the bottom of a container. He used his appliance to make soda fountain drinks. In 1935, Fred Osius improved on Poplawski's idea and invented the famous Waring Blender.

Espresso

Espresso consumption has grown tremendously in the last decade or two. There are drive-through espresso shops in parking lots. Sometimes an espresso cart will just park on the sidewalk, like the hot-dog vendors in cities. People have been buying espresso machines for their homes, too. These machines are smaller than the commercial machines found in cafes, but they work on the same principles. If you go to a cafe or espresso bar and ask for an espresso, what you will get is a shot-sized glass holding a small amount of very strong coffee.

There are many different types of espresso drinks, including cappuccino, cafe latte and cafe mocha. All are made with one or more shots of espresso. A shot of espresso is made by forcing about 1.5 ounces of hot water through tightly packed, finely ground espresso coffee. If everything goes well, what comes out is a dark brown, slightly thick liquid with a small amount of crema (a foam, sort of like the head on a beer) on top. There are many variables in the process of making a shot of espresso. The temperature of the water, the pressure of the water, the fineness of the ground coffee and how tightly the coffee is packed are just a few.

The skilled espresso maker, or barista, controls all of these variables to produce a quality shot of espresso. Let's start with one of the most crucial variables: the coffee. Espresso coffee is a blend of several different types of coffee beans from different countries. The beans are roasted until they are dark and oily-looking.

To force the water through the coffee, the simplest espresso machines use pressure that comes from heating water inside a sealed vessel. These types of machines can be bought for around $50, and there's even one that is made especially to take on a camping trip. They all work on the same principle, so we'll take a look at one of the camping-style machines. In this type of machine, the coffee is packed into a funnel-shaped piece of metal that has a tube extending to the bottom of the reservoir. A few ounces of water are put into the reservoir and the top is screwed on.

When the water is heated over a fire, pressure builds inside the vessel, and the only way for it to escape is up the tube, through the coffee and out of the tube in the top. Since the end of the tube is under water, the pressure forces the hot water up through the tube. There are some disadvantages to a machine like this. The pressure in the system depends on the temperature of the water. The temperature required to build up enough pressure to force the water through the coffee might exceed the ideal brewing temperature.

Coffee Makers

A modern drip coffee maker is a surprisingly simple device. Manufacturers have had 25 years to hone their designs, so these coffee makers are pretty straightforward once you open them up. The heating element is an aluminum extrusion with two parts: a resistive heating element and a tube for water to flow through. The resistive heating element is simply a coiled wire, very similar to the filament of a light bulb or the element in an electric toaster, that gets hot when you run electricity through it. In a resistive element like this, the coil is embedded in a plaster to make it more rugged. The heating element has two jobs:

— When you first put the water in the coffee maker, the heating element boils it.

— Once the coffee is made, the heating element keeps the coffee warm.

The heating element presses directly against the underside of the warming plate, and a white, heat-conductive grease makes sure that the heat transfers efficiently to the plate. This grease, by the way, is extremely messy. You find this grease in all sorts of devices, including stereo amplifiers, power supplies — pretty much anything that has to dissipate heat. The coffee maker's switch turns power to the heating element on and off. To keep the heating element from overheating, there are three solid-state temperature sensors.

The device attached directly to the coil is the primary temperature sensor. When it detects the coil getting too hot, it cuts off the current. Then, when it cools down, it turns the coil back on. By cycling on and off like this, it keeps the coil at an even temperature. The other two devices appear to be thermal fuses. They simply cut power if they sense too high a temperature. They are there for safety reasons, in the event that the main sensor fails. One part that is not visible in this coffee maker is a one-way valve. This valve is either in the hole in the bucket or in the aluminum heating pipe.

If there were no one-way valve, then the boiling water would be just as likely to flow back into the bucket as to rise up the black tube. The one-way valve lets cold water into the aluminum tube, but forces the bubbles of boiling water to flow up the black tube. If you blow on the tube leading into this value, the valve should be open. If you inhale through the tube, the one-way valve should block any air.

Toasters

For lots of people, the toaster is a daily part of breakfast (and lunch and maybe even dinner). A toaster is a machine for toasting food such as sliced bread and bagels. Toasted bread is called toast. Other toastable products may be described as toaster pastry. A typical toaster uses infrared radiation to heat a piece of bread. The heat is usually produced by conducting electricity through nichrome wires (Joule heating).

The toasting process consists of reducing the bread's water content (originally ~35% of total weight), raising its temperature, and slightly charring and caramelising its surface. The caramelisation process is a chemical reaction in which the complex starch molecules break apart into simpler sugar molecules upon heating. That is why toast is usually sweeter than normal bread.

Toaster ovens perform toasting functions of a pop-up toaster, however, the heating elements are positioned horizontally. A toaster oven usually has a glass door and a pull out tray upon which the object to be toasted is placed. Because of its design, a toaster oven can also perform some of the functions provided by a regular oven, but on a somewhat smaller scale. Toaster ovens are freestanding units, commonly placed on countertops or hung from cupboards (kitchen cabinets).

Refrigerators

A refrigerator (often shortened to fridge) or freezer is an electrical appliance that uses refrigeration to help preserve food. An industrial refrigerator or industrial freezer is simply a refrigerator used in an industrial setting, usually in a restaurant or supermarket. They may consist of either a cooling compartment only (a larger refrigerator) or a freezing compartment only (a freezer) or contain both. The dual compartment was introduced commercially by General Electric in 1939. Some refrigerators are now divided into four zones for the storage of different types of food:

— –18°C (0°F) (freezer)

— 0°C (32°F) (meats)

— 4°C (40°F) (refrigerator)

Tips for Personal Hygiene

The first part of sanitation involves your own personal hygiene:

— Don't handle food when you are sick.

— Cover cuts, burns, sores, and abrasions with a tight, dry, antiseptic bandage.

— Shower or bathe daily when you are handling food.

— Keep your clothes clean; wear an apron and change it if you wipe your hands on it or it becomes soiled.

— Keep your hair clean and tied back.

— Use soap and plenty of hot water to wash your hands frequently, especially after any act that might contaminate foods.

Touching your eyes, mouth, ears, nose or hair, smoking, eating or drinking, using the rest room, sneezing or coughing, using a tissue or handkerchief, handling raw food (such as unwashed fruits or vegetables or uncooked meat), taking out the trash, touching a pet or animal, or touching any dirty surfaces (such as wash cloths, money or credit cards, or soiled dishes or linen). If you wear food handler gloves, throw them away after each use, or wash your gloved hands as thoroughly as you would wash your bare hands. Gloves can spread germs just as easily as bare hands.

As you prepare food:

- — Keep raw food away from ready-to-eat or cooked food.
- — Keep all food away from chemicals.
- — Keep cold or frozen foods out of the refrigerator or freezer for as short a time as possible.
- — Wash all raw fruits and vegetables before preparation.
- — Cover food during preparation.
- — When plating food, avoid handling tableware that may touch people's mouths.
- — Never plate food that has touched the floor, unwashed hands, or dirty equipment.
- — Always use tongs or scoops when necessary. Wear latex gloves, and never touch prepared food with your hands.
- — Wipe up spills promptly.
- — Hold food at proper temperatures. Some safe holding temperatures for food are:
- — Stuffed meats and reheated leftovers: 165 degrees Fahrenheit (74 degrees Celsius) or above
- — Cold food: 40 degrees Fahrenheit (4 degrees Celsius) or below
- — Beef and other hot food: 140 degrees Fahrenheit (60 degrees Celsius) or above
- — Fish and poultry: 145 degrees Fahrenheit (63 degrees Celsius) or above
- — Cooked pork, pork products, hamburgers, and eggs: 155 degrees Fahrenheit (68 degrees Celsius)

Clean and sanitise equipment and utensils after each changed use. This includes knives, cutting boards, and thermometers. Storing food properly is also important:

— Do not refreeze food after it has thawed.
— Always label and date leftovers
— Store raw or thawing meats on the lowest refrigerator shelves
— Store shellfish in the original containers
— Always store food in food-grade containers and food wrap

Most harmful germs thrive in temperatures between 40 and 140 degrees Fahrenheit (4 and 60 degrees Celsius). This is known as the Temperature Danger Zone. However, that number may vary slightly as different health departments vary that amount by plus or minus 5 degrees. When you prepare food, keep it out of the Temperature Danger Zone as much as possible. Note that the Temperature Danger Zone includes room temperature. Whenever a potentially hazardous food (fish, beef, poultry, eggs, dairy products, shellfish, pork, some beans) has been in the Temperature Danger Zone for four hours or more, it should be thrown out.

Salmonella bacteria are the number one cause of foodborne infection in the United States. Typical sources of salmonella are meat, poultry, and eggs. Infection can be prevented by cooking food thoroughly and chilling leftovers rapidly. There are two special methods that can help raise the standards of sanitation in your kitchen. The first is the two-spoon tasting method. Use a clean spoon to scoop up the item you wish to taste. Pour that food into a second clean spoon and then taste it.

Never taste food over an open container. This ensures that the spoon you taste from does not go back into the food you are preparing. The second method is also one of the most effective ways of preventing the spread of germs: hand washing. Wet your hands with hot water and wash your hands and wrists with soap for at least 20 seconds.

Scrub your nails with a nail brush. Rinse your hands with hot water for 20 seconds. Follow this procedure twice after using the restroom.

Dry your hands using a single-use paper towel or an air dryer. Kitchen towels can retain germs. The methods you use for thawing food is also an integral part of safe food handling. There are three safe ways of thawing frozen food: in a refrigerator, under running water, and in a microwave. Never thaw frozen food at room temperature. It runs the risk of contamination whenever it is left at room temperature. When thawing frozen food in the refrigerator, remove the food from the freezer. Thaw only the amount of food you need.

Place the wrapped food in a shallow container on the lowest shelf of the refrigerator. Do not unwrap the food for thawing. Make sure the refrigerator temperature is cold enough to keep the thawing food cooler than 40 degrees Fahrenheit (4 degrees Celsius). Leave the food in the refrigerator until it is totally thawed. Large amounts of food or food in boxes can take several days to fully thaw in the refrigerator. When thawing frozen foods under running water, begin by removing only the amount of food you need from the freezer.

Make sure the food is tightly wrapped or placed in a watertight container. Place the wrapped food or container under cold running water of 70 degrees Fahrenheit or less. Make sure the water doesn't directly touch the food and that the food doesn't directly touch the sink. Leave the food under running water until it is completely thawed.

Adjust the microwave setting according to the manufacturer's instructions. Start the microwave. Thaw food in a microwave oven only in emergencies. Cook food immediately after microwave thawing. Microwave cooking causes food to lose moisture and reduces its quality.

4

Food Hygiene during Service

If you have a number of errands to run in addition to shopping for food, be sure to make the grocery store your last stop. If possible, keep a cooler in your car for transporting refrigerated or frozen items. Take food items home immediately and put them in your refrigerator or freezer. Never leave food in a hot vehicle. Check use-by dates and make sure you can use the food by those dates.

Hygiene during Storage

Make sure the food items you buy are in good condition. Refrigerated food should be cold to the touch. Frozen foods should be solid. Canned goods should not be dented, cracked or bulging. Produce should appear fresh. Meat should have a good color and be firm to the touch.

To keep bacteria from rapidly reproducing, be sure your refrigerator is set at the proper temperature. To keep bacteria in check, the refrigerator should run at 40 degrees F, the freezer unit at 0 degrees F. A good general rule to follow is to keep the refrigerator as cold as possible without freezing milk or lettuce. If you don't plan to use it within a few days, freeze fresh meat, poultry or fish. When refrigerating raw meat, poultry or fish, be sure to place the package on a plate so that their juices do not drip on other food. Raw juices can contain bacteria. Always keep eggs in the refrigerator.

Dry Storage of Goods

All canned foods and dry ingredients are stored in a designated area. Foods should not be stored in areas such as restrooms, furnace rooms, stairwells or hallways. Foods should be stored off the floor and in closed containers. Storage areas should be well ventilated and pest free. Dry storage areas can become a food source for rodent and insects. Keeping containers closed, in sound condition and off the floor help to keep the storage area pest free. Stock rotation is a good management practice. Foods and chemicals need to be stored separately. Chemicals should be stored below and away from foods to prevent chemical contamination.

Cold Holding of Food

Cold holding is storing food under refrigeration at 41°F or below. Refrigeration prevents food from becoming a hazard by slowing the growth of most microbes. Some organisms like Listeria monocytogenes is significantly slowed but not stopped by refrigeration.

Walk-in Refrigerator Temperature

The walk-in refrigerator is the major cold storage area in a food service establishment. The temperature of a walk-in refirgerator must be sufficient to adequately hold the food temperature at 41°F or below. The temperature of a walk-in refrigerator is usually colder than 41°F. to compensate the opening and closing of doors and demands of adding additional foods for storage and cooling. Foods need to be stored to prevent contamination. All cooked foods and foods that will receive no further cooking should be stored above other foods. Foods need to be stored to allow enough space for air to circulate around them.

Hygiene during Preparation

Be sure to wash your hands in warm soapy water before preparing food and after using the bathroom, changing diapers and handling pets. Kitchen towels, sponges and cloths can harbor bacteria. Wash them often and replace sponges every few weeks. Keep raw meat, poultry and fish and their juices away from other food. For example, after cutting up meat or poultry, be sure to wash your hands, the knife and the cutting board in hot soapy water before you start to dice salad ingredients. Thaw food in the microwave or in the refrigerator. Do not thaw items on the kitchen counter. This allows bacteria to grow in the outer layers of the food before the inside thaws. If you plan to marinate food, do it in the refrigerator, too.

Thorough cooking kills harmful bacteria. If you eat meat, poultry, fish, oysters or eggs that are raw or only partially cooked, you may be exposing yourself to bacteria that can make you ill. This is particularly important for children, pregnant women, the elderly, and those whose immune systems are compromised by illness or by medical treatment (for example, chemotherapy). Use a meat thermometer to ensure that meat and poultry are cooked to the appropriate temperature.

Salmonella, a bacteria that causes food poisoning, can grow inside fresh, unbroken eggs. Be sure to cook eggs until the yolk and white are firm, not runny. Scramble eggs to a firm texture. Avoid recipes in which eggs remain raw or only partially cooked (for example, mousse, egg drinks, Caesar salad, etc.). Pasteurized eggs or egg substitute can be used instead. If you prepare and cook food ahead of time, divide large portions into small, shallow containers and refrigerate. This ensures rapid, safe cooling.

While microwaves are great time savers, they can leave cold spots in food. Bacteria can survive in these spots. Be sure to cover food with a lid or plastic wrap so steam can help to promote thorough cooking. Vent plastic wrap and make sure it doesn't touch the food. Stir and rotate food for even cooking. If your microwave does not have a turntable, rotate the dish by hand once or twice during the cooking time. Observe the standing time called for in a recipe or on package directions. During the standing time, the food finishes cooking. Use an oven temperature probe or a meat thermometer to check that food is done. Be sure to check several spots.

Thawing Foods

Thawing foods may take several hours or days depending on the size of the food item being thawed. Thawing must be done so that the risk of cross-contamination is reduced, and the time that potentially hazardous food is in the temperature danger zone (41°F to 140°F) is kept to minimum. To thaw food safely:

— Thaw under refrigeration (41°F and below)

— Under cold running potable water (safe to drink) of 70°F or less as part of the cooking process.

— In a microwave then transferred to conventional cooking equipment with no interruption in the process.

Cooking Temperatures

Cooking is the thermal heating of foods at sufficent temperature over time to kill microorganisms in the food. The following are the requirements for the different foods:

Beef, fish, seafood, eggs	145°F.
Rare Roast Beef	130°F.
Pork	145°F.

Poultry, food containing poultry, stuffed meats or stuffing containing meat, casseroles, containing potentially hazardous foods	165°F.
Restructed meat, ground or fabricated meat	155°F.

Cooking requirements are based on the biology of pathogens. Different species of microorganisms have different susceptibilities to heat. Food characteristics also contribute to the lethality of cooking temperatures. Heat penetrates different foods at different rates. High fat content reduces the lethality of heat. High humidity in the cooking container or the moisture content of the food aid the lethality of heat.

To effectively eliminate pathogens, there are a number of factors to consider: the level of pathogens in the raw product and the initial temperature of the food and the bulk of the food. Another factor to consider, to kill the pathogenic organisms in food, cooking must heat all parts of the food to the required temperatures.

Reheating

Bring sauces, soups and gravies to a boil. Heat other leftovers thoroughly to 165 degrees F. Microwave leftovers using a lid or vented plastic wrap to ensure thorough heating.

Hot Holding Foods

Once a food is heated or cooked, the food must be maintained at a temperature to limit the growth of bacteria. The correct hot holding temperature is 140°F. The potential for growth of pathogenic bacteria increases once a food is reheated than the potential in raw foods. The spoilage organisms that may be present in raw foods inhibit the growth of pathogenic organisms by competition. Once a food is cooked, these spoilage organisms are reduced.

Cooling Foods

Cooling is a process of removing heat from food quickly enough to prevent microbial growth. One method is done by placing foods in shallow containers no deeper than 2 inches and leaving them uncovered until cold, 41°F or below. When potentially hazardous food is cooled for an extended period, the food is subject to the growth of a variety of pathogenic micro-organisms. Bacteria grow ideally between 70—120°F. (The human body temperature falls in this range). The longer the time the food is allowed to be held in this range, the greater the risk of microbial growth. Excessive time for cooling potentially hazard food has consistently been identified as one of the leading contributing factors to foodborne illness.

Cross-contamination

Bacteria (pathogens) can be transferred to food from utensils, surfaces (cutting boards), food workers hands, raw meats, poultry, fish and seafood. Contamination is the presence of disease-causing microorganisms or harmful substances in food. Food can become contaminated at any time and can be contaminated by other foods. To help prevent cross-contamination, raw meats, fish, and poultry must be kept away from cooked and ready-to-eat foods. (i.e. separate cutting boards, separation of duties, preparing vegetables before preparing meats.) Employees need to minimise bare hand contact with cooked and ready-to-eat foods.

Room Temperature Storage

Temperature is one of the prime factors that control the growth of bacteria in food. Many types of pathogens and spoilage bacteria are prevented from multiplying to significant levels that cause foodborne illness with proper holding practices. All foods need to be stored cold 41°F and below or hot 140°F or above. Preparation procedures should have built in barriers to limit the time potentially hazardous foods are in the temperature danger zone. (41°F to 140°F.) Control measure to ensure foods are out of temperature for limited times include:

- Refrigerate foods before preparation.
- Prepare foods not further in advance than necessary.
- Prepare small batches of food and return them to the refrigerator before cooking and serving.

Final Cook Temperatures

Cooking requirements are based on the biology of pathogens. The amount of heat required to destroy the organisms will vary. Different species of microorganisms are susceptable to varied levels of heat. To kill all pathogens in foods, cooking must bring all parts of the food to required temperature for a correct length of time.

Hygiene during Serving

Never leave perishable food unrefrigerated for more than two hours. Bacteria that can cause food poisoning grow quickly at warm temperatures. Always use clean dishes and utensils to serve food, not those you used to prepare the food. If you grill food, serve it on a clean plate, not on the one that held the raw meat, poultry or fish. Pack lunches in insulated carriers with a cold pack. Be sure your children know not to leave lunches in direct sunlight or on warm radiators.

Carry picnic food in a cooler with a cold pack. Try to keep the cooler in the shade and do not open the lid any more than is necessary. If you have a party, keep cold food on ice or keep refrigerated until time to replenish platters. If serving hot food, maintain it at 140 degrees F or divide into smaller serving platters, which can be refrigerated until time to warm them up for serving.

Serving Size

The serving size refers to the average amount or portion size that a person eats at one time. If the portion of the food that you eat is more or less than the serving size, then you need to adjust the nutrient and calorie values. For example, if you eat twice the amount listed in the serving size, then you must double the nutrient and calorie values. Conversely, the portion size for younger children is likely to be less than the serving size. If your preschool age child eats a portion that is one-half the serving size, then cut the nutrient and calorie values in half too.

If you eat the whole package or container of food, which has four servings, then you must multiply nutrient and calorie values by four. Refers to the number of nutrients and calories for each serving of food. A common mistake that people make is to just look at the calorie and nutrient information and not take into account how many servings are in the container. In the above example, if you eat the whole container of food, you might think you were only consuming 90 calories, but the whole container actually contained 4 servings, which would equal 360 calories.

Calories

Refers to the number of calories for each serving of food. Again, take into account how many servings you have had when determining how many calories you have eaten.

The percent daily value for fat, cholesterol, carbohydrate, sodium, potassium and protein are based on a 2,000 calorie diet. These values may be higher or lower depending on the amount of calories in your diet. Your diet each day should reach 100% for total carbohydrate, dietary fiber, vitamins and minerals.

Handling Leftovers

Divide large amounts of leftovers into small, shallow containers for quick cooling in the refrigerator. Don't pack the refrigerator; cool air must be able to circulate to keep food safe. With poultry or other stuffed meats, remove stuffing and refrigerate it in a separate container.

Personal Hygiene in the Kitchen

As your hands are often in direct contact with food they are one of the main routes for contaminating food and transferring food poisoning bacteria. All those handling food must wash their hands—before handling any food or equipment. After handling raw meat and chicken and before you handle other foods. Immediately after going to the toilet, blowing your nose, coughing, sneezing, smoking and handling waste food or rubbish.

All those handling food must:

- Avoid unnecessarily handling food, but should use tongs, forks, spoons, scoops, or other suitable utensils where possible.
- Use a clean spoon to sample food, not your fingers.
- Not cough or sneeze over or around food.
- Not smoke while preparing or handling food.
- Keep all utensils, cutting boards, stove tops, fridges, and benches clean.

— Use only clean dish cloths and tea towels.
— Avoid handling the food contact surfaces of crockery and cutlery.
— Throw out chipped or cracked crockery.
— Cover any cuts or sores on your hands with a bandage, or use plastic gloves.
— Not use the kitchen sink for washing your pet's dishes, or washing babies' nappies or clothes.

When shopping

— Shop only at hygienic shops.
— Demand hygienic service.
— Only buy High Risk Foods that are refrigerated.
— Insist on tongs.
— Don't finger food.
— Replace food covers.
— Don't cough over food.
— Keep children from touching food.
— Leave animals outside.
— Don't litter.

High Risk Foods

High risk foods are those perishable foods which can support the growth of harmful bacteria and are intended to be eaten without further treatment such as cooking, which would destroy such organisms. They include;

— All cooked meat and poultry.
— Cooked meat products including gravy, stock, and roll/sandwich fillings.
— Milk, cream, artificial cream, custards and dairy products.

— Cooked eggs and products made with eggs, eg mayonnaise.

— Shellfish and other seafood.

— Cooked rice.

Don't leave High Risk Foods sitting at room temperature. Unfortunately contaminated food usually looks, tastes, and smells completely normal, and cannot be detected without laboratory examination.

Process Approach to Food Service

When conducting the hazard analysis, food manufacturers usually use food commodities as an organisational tool and follow the flow of one product. This is a very useful approach for producers or processors since they are usually handling one product at a time. By contrast, in retail and food service operations, foods of all types are worked together to produce the final product. This makes a different approach to the hazard analysis necessary.

Conducting the hazard analysis by using the food preparation processes common to a specific operation is often more efficient and useful for retail and food service operators. This is called the "Process Approach". The process approach can best be described as dividing the many food flows in an establishment into broad categories based on activities or stages in the flow of food through your establishment, then analysing the hazards, and placing managerial controls on each grouping.

Flow of food

The flow of food in a retail or food service establishment is the path that food follows from receiving through service or sale to the consumer. Several activities or stages make up the flow of food and are called operational steps. Examples of operational steps include receiving, storing, preparing, cooking, cooling, reheating, holding, assembling, packaging, serving, and selling. Keep in mind that the terminology used for operational steps may differ between food service and retail food store operations.

Foods that go through the danger zone only once are classified as Same Day Service, while foods that go through more than once are classified as Complex food preparation.

The three food preparation processes conducted in retail and food service establishments are not intended to be all-inclusive. For instance, quick service facilities may have "cook and serve" processes specific to their operation. These processes are likely to be different from the "Same Day Service" preparation processes in full service restaurants since many of their foods are generally cooked and hot held before service. In addition, in retail food stores, operational steps such as packaging and assembly may be included in all of the food preparation processes prior to being sold to the consumer.

It is also very common for a retail or food service operator to have a single menu item (i.e. chicken salad sandwich) that is created by combining several components produced using more than one kind of food preparation process. It is important for you to remember that even though variations of the three food preparation process flows are common, the control measures — actions or activities that can be used to prevent, eliminate, or reduce food safety hazards — to be implemented in each process will generally be the same based on the number of times the food goes through the temperature danger zone.

In the "process approach", conducting a hazard analysis on individual food items is time and labor intensive and is generally unnecessary. An establishment has dozens of food items (including baked chicken and meatloaf) in the "Preparation for Same Day Service" category. Each of the food items may have unique hazards, but regardless of their individual hazards, control via proper cooking and holding will generally ensure the safety of all of the foods in this category.

In developing your food safety management system, keep in mind that active managerial control of risk factors common to each process can be achieved by either designating certain operational steps as critical control points (CCPs) or by implementing prerequisite programmes. In combination with prerequisite programmes, will constitute a complete food safety management system.

Facility-wide considerations

In order to have active managerial control over personal hygiene and cross-contamination, you must implement certain control measures in all phases of your operation. All of the following control measures should be implemented regardless of the food preparation process used:

— No bare hand contact with ready-to-eat foods (or use of an approved, alternative procedure) to help prevent the transfer of viruses, bacteria, or parasites from hands

— Proper handwashing to help prevent the transfer of viruses, bacteria, or parasites from hands to food

— Restriction or exclusion of ill employees to help prevent the transfer of viruses, bacteria, or parasites from hands to food

— Prevention of cross-contamination of ready-to-eat food or clean and sanitised food-contact surfaces with soiled cutting boards, utensils, aprons, etc. or raw animal foods

Several food flows are represented by particular process. Many of these food flows are common to both retail food stores and food service facilities, while others only apply to retail operations. Raw, ready-to-eat food like sashimi, raw oysters, and salads are grouped in this category. Components of these foods are received raw and will not be cooked prior to consumption.

Foods cooked at the processing level but that undergo no further cooking at the retail level before being consumed are also represented in this category. Examples of these kinds of foods are deli meats, cheeses, and other pasteurised products. In addition, foods that are received and sold raw but are to be cooked by the consumer after purchase, i.e. hamburger meat, chicken, and steaks, are also included in this category.

All the foods in this category lack a kill (cook) step while at the retail or food service establishment. In other words, there is no complete trip made through the danger zone for the purpose of destroying pathogens. You can ensure that the food received in your establishment is as safe as possible by requiring purchase specifications. Without a kill step to destroy pathogens, your primary responsibility will be to prevent further contamination by ensuring that your employees follow good hygienic practices.

Cross-contamination must be prevented by properly storing your products away from raw animal foods and soiled equipment and utensils. Foodborne illness may result from ready-to-eat food being held at unsafe temperatures for long periods of time due to the outgrowth of bacteria. In addition to the facility-wide considerations, a food safety management system involving this food preparation process should focus on ensuring that you have active managerial control over the following:

— Cold holding or using time alone to inhibit bacterial growth and toxin production.

— Food source (especially for shellfish due to concerns with viruses, natural toxins, and Vibrio and for certain marine finfish intended for raw consumption due to concerns with ciguatera toxin).

— Receiving temperatures (especially certain species of marine finfish due to concerns with scombrotoxin)

— Date marking of ready-to-eat PHF held for more than 24 hours to control the growth of Listeria monocytogenes.

— Freezing certain species of fish intended for raw consumption due to parasite concerns.

— Cooling from ambient temperature to prevent the outgrowth of spore-forming or toxin-forming bacteria

In this food preparation process, food passes through the danger zone only once in the retail or food service establishment before it is served or sold to the consumer. Food is usually cooked and held hot until served, i.e. fried chicken, but can also be cooked and served immediately. In addition to the facility-wide considerations, a food safety management system involving this food preparation process should focus on ensuring that you have active managerial control over the following:

— Cooking to destroy bacteria and parasites

— Hot holding or using time alone to prevent the outgrowth of spore-forming bacteria

Approved food source, proper receiving temperatures, and proper cold holding prior to cooking are also important if dealing with certain marine finfish due to concerns with ciguatera toxin and scombrotoxin.

Foods prepared in large volumes or in advance for next day service usually follow an extended process flow.

These foods pass through the temperature danger zone more than one time; thus, the potential for the growth of spore-forming or toxigenic bacteria is greater in this process. Failure to adequately control food product temperatures is one of the most frequently encountered risk factors contributing to foodborne illness. In addition, foods in this category have the potential to be recontaminated with L. monocytogenes, which could grow during refrigerated storage. Food handlers minimise the time foods are at unsafe temperatures.

In addition to the facility-wide considerations, a food safety management system involving this food preparation process should focus on ensuring that you have active managerial control over the following:

— Cooking to destroy bacteria and parasites

— Cooling to prevent the outgrowth of spore-forming or toxin-forming bacteria

— Hot and cold holding or using time alone to inhibit bacterial growth and toxin formation

— Date marking of ready-to-eat PHF held for more than 24 hours to control the growth of Listeria monocytogenes

— Reheating for hot holding, if applicable

Approved food source, proper receiving temperatures, and proper cold holding prior to cooking are also important if dealing with certain marine finfish due to concerns with ciguatera toxin and scombrotoxin.

Food Safety

The goal of a food safety management system is to control certain factors that lead to out-of-control hazards. Because many foods are agricultural products and have started their journey to your door as animals and plants raised in the environment, they may contain microscopic organisms.

Some of these organisms are pathogens which means that under the right conditions and in the right numbers, they can make someone who eats them sick. Raw animal foods such as meat, poultry, fish, shellfish, and eggs often carry bacteria, viruses, or parasites that can be harmful to humans. Food can become contaminated by toxic chemicals or toxins in your establishment or in the environment. Physical objects may also contaminate food and cause injury. Food may become naturally contaminated from the soil in which it is grown or from harvest, storage, or transportation practices.

Some foods undergo further processing and at times, despite best efforts, become contaminated. These inherent hazards, along with the hazards that may be introduced in your establishment such as metal fragments from grinding can lead to injury, illness, or death. Hazards are a huge threat to your business. Think of hazards as ticking bombs in your establishment.

Hazards include:-

- Biological agents
    - Bacteria and their toxins
    - Parasites
    - Viruses
- Physical Objects
    - Bandages
    - Jewelry
    - Stones
    - Glass
    - Bone and metal fragments
    - Packaging materials
- Chemical Contamination
    - Natural plant and animal toxins

— Unlabeled allergens (allergen-causing protein)
— Nonfood-grade lubricants
— Cleaning compounds
— Food additives
— Insecticides

Active Managerial Control

The term "active managerial control" is used to describe your role for developing and implementing a food safety management system to reduce the occurrence of risk factors. Although the term "active managerial control" may be new to some, the basic management principles are probably already being used in your day-to-day operations.

Active managerial control means the purposeful incorporation of specific actions or procedures by industry management into the operation of your business to attain control over foodborne illness risk factors. It embodies a preventive rather than reactive approach to food safety. Having active managerial control includes having procedures in place for controlling identified foodborne illness risk factors through a continuous system of monitoring and verification.

There are many management systems that you can voluntarily implement to achieve active managerial control of risk factors. Effective elements of a food safety management system are

— Certified food protection managers who have shown a proficiency of required information by passing a test that is part of an accredited programme
— Standard operating procedures (SOPs) for performing critical operational steps in a food preparation process such as cooling

- Recipe cards that contain the specific steps for preparing a food item and the food safety critical limits such as final cooking temperatures that need to be monitored and verified
- Purchase specifications
- Equipment and facility design and maintenance
- Monitoring procedures
- Record keeping
- Employee health policy for restricting or excluding ill employees
- Manager and employee training
- On-going quality control and assurance
- Specific goal-oriented plans, like Risk Control Plans (RCPs), that outline procedures for controlling specific foodborne illness risk factors

Developing Food Safety System

The owner, the managers, chefs, cooks, dishwashers, wait staff, and other individuals who might be actively involved in the preparation and service of the food. Although managers are responsible for designing the system, implementation involves the efforts and commitment of every employee.

Training managers and employees in their respective roles is crucial to the success of your food safety management system. You may consider working with outside consultants, industry trade associations, university extension services, and your regulatory authority to ensure that your food safety management system is based on the best available science and that it will control the identified hazards.

Just like a well-played chess game, building a food safety management system takes time, patience, and determination. Careful consideration must be given to all aspects of your operation affecting food safety. To assist you in building your food safety management system, a series of procedural steps have been developed to guide you through the process.

Prerequisite programmes

If you want to build a sturdy home, you should start with a strong foundation. The same is true of a food safety management system. In order for your food safety management system to be effective, you should first develop and implement a strong foundation of procedures that address the basic operational and sanitation conditions within your operation. These procedures are collectively termed "prerequisite programmes."

When prerequisite programmes are in place, you can focus more attention on the hazards associated with the food and its preparation. Before beginning to write your food safety management system, it is recommended that you develop and implement prerequisite programmes. Prerequisite programmes may include such things as:-

— Vendor certification programmes
— Training programmes
— Allergen management
— Buyer specifications
— Recipe/process instructions
— First-In-First-Out (FIFO) procedures
— Other Standard Operating Procedures (SOPs)

Basic prerequisite programmes should be in place to:-

— Protect products from contamination by biological, chemical, and physical food safety hazards

— Control bacterial growth that can result from temperature abuse
— Maintain equipment

Control Contamination of Food. These procedures insure that:-

— Soiled and unsanitised surfaces of equipment and utensils do not contact raw or cooked (ready-to-eat) food
— Workers with certain symptoms, such as vomiting or diarrhea, are restricted or excluded
— Raw animal foods do not contaminate cooked (ready-to-eat) food
— Effective handwashing is practiced
— Eating, smoking, and drinking in food preparation areas are prohibited
— Water in contact with food and food-contact surfaces and used in the manufacture of ice is potable
— Toxic compounds are properly labeled, stored, and safely used
— Contaminants such as condensate, lubricants, pesticides, cleaning compounds, sanitising agents, and additional toxic materials do not contact food, food-packaging materials, and food-contact surfaces
— Food, food-packaging materials, and food-contact surfaces are not contaminated by physical hazards such as broken glass from light fixtures, jewelry, etc.
— An effective pest control system is in place
— Hair restraints are used
— Clean clothing is worn
— The wearing of jewelry (other than a wedding ring) is prohibited

Control Bacterial Growth: These procedures ensure that all potentially hazardous food is received and stored at a refrigerated temperature of 41°F or below. Note that the Food Code makes some allowances for specific foods that may be received at higher temperatures.

Prerequisite Programmes to Maintain Equipment. These procedures ensure that:-

- — Food-contact surfaces, including utensils, are cleaned, sanitised, and maintained in good condition
- — Temperature measuring devices (e.g., thermometer or temperature recording device) are calibrated regularly
- — Cooking and hot holding equipment (grills, ovens, steam tables, conveyer cookers, etc.) are routinely checked, calibrated, and operated to ensure correct product temperature
- — Cold holding and cooling equipment (refrigerators, rapid chill units, freezers, salad bars, etc.) are routinely checked, calibrated, and operated to ensure correct product temperature
- — Warewashing equipment is operated according to manufacturer's specifications
- — Toilet facilities are accessible to employees and maintained

The items addressed by this procedural step are the foundation by which your entire food safety management system is based. The success of any food safety management system is dependent on how well you control these basic sanitation issues in your establishment.

With this in mind, consider how you can actively monitor the activities associated with the prerequisite programmes to ensure that they are being implemented properly. If you decide to control certain items in your food safety management system through prerequisite programmes, monitoring of the programmes is recommended. If you see areas needing improvement, you should take corrective actions immediately.

Grouping menu items

To begin grouping your menu items/products, you should review how your menu items or products flow through your operation. You should note whether they undergo a cook step for same day service, receive additional cooling and reheating following a cook step, or have no cook step involved. Looking at your menu or food list, you should place each item into the appropriate food preparation process. You may discover that more than one food preparation process is conducted within your operation.

Food safety hazards

In developing a food safety management system, you should identify the food safety hazards that exist in the flow of food in your operation from receiving to service or sale. By identifying the food safety hazards present in your system, you should then be able to determine the possible control measures that may be implemented to achieve active managerial control of the foodborne illness risk factors leading to out-of-control hazards. Control measures are any actions or activities that can be used to prevent, eliminate, or reduce an identified hazard.

The specific food safety hazards for each of the products within a particular food preparation process may be varied, but the recommended control measures for each of the products in each process will generally be the same. As you conduct the hazard analysis, you will most likely find that regardless of the specific food safety hazards present in the products in any particular food preparation process, the foods within each of the food preparation processes share common categories of hazards.

This is why the control measures you apply to the products in each of the three food preparation processes will generally be the same. Because of this, you may use general categories to designate the types of food safety hazards present in your operation. You may have baked chicken, fried fish, grilled hamburgers, and baked meatloaf that are all cooked and hot held before service. While each of these foods may have unique food safety hazards, they all share general categories of hazards and therefore the control measures that you may implement are basically the same.

Vegetative bacteria are controlled through proper cooking, spore-forming or toxin-forming bacteria are controlled through proper hot holding, and fecal-oral route pathogens such as Shigella, Salmonellae, and viruses are controlled through good hygienic practices such as proper handwashing, no bare hand contact with ready-to-eat food, and implementation of employee health policies. In addition, pathogens resulting from cross-contamination may be controlled by proper sanitisation and storage practices.

The Food Code provides specific measurable criteria referred to as critical limits designed to prevent, eliminate, or reduce hazards in foods. The critical limits are based on the best available science and pertain to control measures applied within operational steps. Common examples might be time/temperature standards and no bare hand contact with ready-to-eat food. You should make sure that you have established the appropriate critical limits to control the identified hazards. It is recommended that you refer to the most recent version of the Food Code or your state, local, or tribal regulations for help with determining the appropriate critical limits for the identified control measures.

Monitoring procedures

Monitoring is observing or measuring specific operational steps in the food process to determine if your critical limits are being met. This activity is recommended to make sure your critical control points are under control. Monitoring will identify when there is a loss of control or a trend toward a loss of control so that corrective actions can be taken.

In your food safety management system, certain processes have been identified as requiring active managerial control. What you are going to monitor depends on the critical limits you have established. Final temperature and time measurements are very important, and you should determine how you will effectively monitor the critical limits for them.

Determining the appropriate means for monitoring is an important factor in developing your food safety management system. If equipment is selected to monitor a specific CCP, you should ensure that it is accurate and routinely calibrated to ensure critical limits are met. The equipment you choose should also be appropriate for the monitoring that is being done. For example, a thermocouple with a thin probe is the most appropriate tool for measuring the final product temperature of thin hamburger patties.

When deciding how often you will monitor, you should ensure that the monitoring interval will be reliable enough to ensure hazards are being controlled. Your procedure for monitoring should be simple and easy to follow. Individuals chosen to be responsible for a monitoring activity may be a manager, line supervisor, or other reliable employee. FDA recommends that employees be given the training and equipment necessary to properly perform the monitoring activities.

Whenever a critical limit is not met, a corrective action must be carried out immediately. A corrective action may be simply continuing to heat food to the required temperature. Other corrective actions may be more complicated, such as rejecting a shipment of raw oysters that does not have the required tags or segregating and holding a product until an evaluation is done.

In the event that a corrective action is taken, you should review and modify your food safety management system, if necessary. Even with the best of systems, errors occur during food storage and preparation. A benefit to both you and your regulator is the ability to show that immediate corrective action was taken to ensure that no unsafe food was served or sold to the consumer. It is important to communicate to management all corrective actions in writing or electronically.

Ongoing verification

Control of food safety practices, implementation of the system should to be verified. Verification is simply making sure that you are performing the activities as described in your food safety management system.

Routine monitoring should not be confused with verification. Verification is making sure that all the activities carried out in the implementation of your food safety management system are being done properly and at the required frequency. Monitoring is one of the many activities that needs to be verified. This is a vital step in ensuring that you have established active managerial control of identified hazards.

Verification should be conducted by someone other than the person who is directly responsible for performing the activities specified in the food safety management system. That person might be a manager, supervisor, designated individual, food safety professional, or even your health inspector. If involved in the verification process, your inspector can offer suggestions for how you can strengthen your food safety management system. Verification activities are conducted frequently, such as daily, weekly, monthly, etc., and may include:-

— Observing that person(s) are carrying out the critical procedures correctly

— Observing the person doing the monitoring and determining whether monitoring is being done as planned

— Reviewing the monitoring records to determine if they are completed accurately and consistently

— Determining whether the records show that the frequency of monitoring stated in the plan is being followed

— Ensuring that corrective action was taken when the person monitoring found and recorded that the critical limit was not met

— Confirming that all equipment, including equipment used for monitoring, was operated, maintained and calibrated properly

Verification should occur at a frequency that can ensure the food safety management system is being followed continuously to:-

— Prevent unsafe food from reaching the consumer

— Take corrective action without loss of product

— Confirm that prescribed personnel practices are followed

— Ensure that personnel have the tools for proper personal hygiene and sanitary practices (e.g., handwashing facilities, sanitising equipment, cleaning supplies, temperature measuring devices, etc.)

— Comply with the established control procedures

Keep records

As the manager of your operation, you may have several duties to perform in addition to making sure that the activities in your food safety management system are being performed at the proper frequency and with the proper method. Documenting these activities provides one mechanism for verifying that the activities were properly completed.

While record keeping is voluntary in most retail and food service operations, maintaining documentation of the activities in your food safety management system may be vital to its success. Remember that by keeping records you are going above and beyond what your regulations normally require. Records provide documentation that appropriate corrective actions were taken when critical limits were not met.

In the event your establishment is implicated in a foodborne illness, documentation of activities related to monitoring and corrective actions can provide proof that reasonable care was exercised in the operation of your establishment. Records may also show that on-going verification was conducted on the food safety management system. In many cases, your records can serve a dual purpose of ensuring quality and food safety.

In order to develop the most effective record keeping system for your operation, you should determine what documented information will assist you in managing the control of food safety hazards. A record keeping system can be simple and needs to be designed to meet the needs of your individual establishment. You do not necessarily need to develop new records to document the actions in the system.

Some recorded information like shellfish tags should already be part of your food safety management system, and an additional record may not be needed. Your record keeping system may use existing paperwork such as delivery invoices for documenting product temperature. Many retail and food service establishments have implemented comprehensive record keeping systems without having to generate a mountain of paperwork

Employees are an important source for developing simple and effective record keeping procedures. You should ask employees how they are currently monitoring CCPs or prerequisite programmes and discuss with them the types of corrective actions they are currently taking when a critical limit is not met. Managers are responsible for designing the system, but effective day-to-day implementation involves every employee.

The simplest record keeping system that lends itself to integration into existing operations is always best. A simple, yet effective, system is easier to use and communicate to your employees. Record keeping systems designed to document process rather than product information may be more useful in a retail and food service establishment, especially if you frequently change menu items or products. Accurately documenting processes like cooking, cooling, and reheating provides a mechanism for ensuring that you have active managerial control of risk factors.

There are at least 5 types of records that may be maintained to support your food safety management system:

— Records documenting the activities related to the prerequisite programmes

— Monitoring records

— Corrective action records

— Verification and validation records

— Calibration records

Once a specific process has been shown to work for you, such as an ice bath method for cooling certain foods, the frequency of record keeping may be modified. This approach is extremely effective for labor-intensive processes related to:-

— Cooking large volumes of food where a temperature check of each individual item is impractical

— Implementing a verified process that will allow employees to complete the procedure in a scheduled workday

— Cooling foods or leftovers at the end of the business day

— Maintaining cold holding temperatures of ready-to-eat, potentially hazardous foods in walk-in refrigeration units

Special Considerations Regarding Records: You are encouraged to periodically obtain feedback from your regulatory authority regarding how well your system is working. You can invite your regulatory authority to review or verify your voluntarily-implemented food safety management system. This allows them the opportunity to offer suggestions for problems that they find in the operation of your system, including discrepancies with the monitoring and record keeping procedures.

Remember that the maintenance of records is required in the Food Code only in a limited number of cases. When your food safety management system is voluntary, their review of your system is by invitation only and they can only document violations that they observe as they would during routine inspections. Records generated in support of a voluntary food safety management systems may not to be used to verify compliance with your regulations unless the records are specifically required by your regulations.

In contrast, if your health inspector finds documented cases of inadequately cooked or hot held foods being sold to consumers, he or she cannot take regulatory action against you based on the documentation. Documentation of hot holding and cooking, like most processes in your regulations, is probably not required. The fact that you are keeping records of these processes means that you are probably going above and beyond what is required by your regulations. Of course, your health inspector may point out discrepancies and offer recommendations to you in hopes of preventing the problems from happening again.

Of course, if during the review of your system evidence is found that a product still in circulation poses a serious health threat to the public, the health inspector may initiate an appropriate regulatory investigation as dictated by your regulatory agency. If it is known by your health inspector or you that a product still on the market poses a health threat to consumers, both of you should play your respective roles to remove the product immediately. This may involve voluntary recall of the suspected products.

Periodic validation

Once your food safety management system is established, you should periodically review it to determine whether the food safety hazards are controlled when the system is implemented properly. This is known as validation.

Changes in suppliers, products, or preparation procedures may prompt a revalidation of your food safety management system. A small change could result in a drastically different outcome from what you expect. You may benefit from both internal (quality assurance) and external validations that may involve assistance from the regulatory authority or other consultants.

Validation is conducted less frequently (e.g., yearly) than on-going verification. It is a review or audit of the plan to determine if:-

— Any new product/processes/menu items have been added to the menu

— Suppliers, customers, equipment, or facilities have changed

— Prerequisite programmes are current and implemented

— Worksheets are still current

— CCPs are still valid, or if new CCPs are needed

— Critical limits are set realistically and are adequate to control the hazard (e.g., the time needed to cook a turkey to meet the Food Code internal temperature requirement)

— Monitoring equipment has been calibrated as planned.

5

Safe Food Storage

Food spoilage occurs primarily through the action of bacteria, molds, and yeasts. Spoilage organisms break down the complex organic substances in foods into their simple, inorganic components. This process is responsible for the changes in the odour, colour, texture, appearance, and taste of food products, which indicate spoilage. Spoiled food is unfit for human consumption.

Many factors contribute to food spoilage. A variety of microorganisms are often involved in the breakdown of organic substances. Enzymatic autolysis accelerates the rate of spoilage. Insects and rodents also damage food products and make them unfit for human consumption. Physical changes (exposure to extreme temperatures or excessive pressure) and careless handling cause bruising. Chemical reactions other than autolysis can also be responsible for food spoilage.

Most food spoilage occurs when foods are at the storing control point. Storage area standards must be designed to prevent or minimise food spoilage and exposure of food products to pathogenic organisms. In general, raw food products can be placed in one of three broad categories-perishable, semi-perishable, non-perishable-based on their susceptibility to microbial spoilage. Perishable food products spoil readily without special processing or preservation techniques. This category includes most products used daily in a food service facility: meats, poultry, fish, shellfish, eggs, dairy products, and most fruits and vegetables. Semiperishable food products have a longer shelf life than perishable foods. These products spoil more slowly when stored under recommended time-temperature combinations. Included in this category are nuts, apples, potatoes, and waxed vegetables such as cucumbers. Non-perishable food products are the most resistant to spoilage unless they are improperly handled and stored. This category includes most dry grocery items, such as sugar, flour, spices, and dry beans. Food preservation methods are designed to increase the shelf life and maintain the desirable physical and chemical properties of food.

Food Preservation Methods

Food processors discovered that one of the best ways to preserve food was to practice strict microbiological control. Along with controlling pathogenic organisms, food processors and manufacturers learned to control organisms responsible for food spoilage. They succeeded in increasing the shelf life and availability of food products for the growing number of city dwellers. In time, processed food products even became popular with farm families. Today food-processing plants use a variety of methods to provide wholesome food products to industrialised world.

In recent years, several self-proclaimed "food experts" have tried to persuade the public that the food supply is loaded with unnecessary levels of food additives. But these food additives control undesirable microbes and increase the availability of food. To condemn food additives without acknowledging their benefits does a disservice to the uninformed consumer. Without such additives, we would be buying food products like those in turn-of-the-century general stores. Few of us would be willing to give up the convenience of modern supermarkets just to avoid additives.

Food additives are already closely regulated in the United States. Unsafe or unapproved food or colour additives may not be incorporated into food products. However, consumer interest in this area is unlikely to diminish. The best protection that a food service operation has is to be informed and to obtain food products only from approved sources.

There are four main objectives of food preservation. Some preservation methods are designed to lengthen the lag phase of bacterial growth. Another objective of food preservation is to delay undesirable autolysis. This is achieved by destroying enzymes or preventing enzymatic action. The third objective is to minimise the damage caused by insects, rodents, and physical trauma. The fourth objective, the prevention of microbiological breakdown of food, is probably the most important. All methods of food preservation are designed to achieve one or more of these objectives.

Low-Temperature Preservation

Low temperatures preserve food products during their flow through the control points of a food service operation. They slow the growth of spoilage organisms and decrease the rate of chemical reactions and enzyme activity. The rate of microbial reproduction decreases as the temperature drops, and eventually stops altogether. Some organisms may survive the low temperatures and form spores which, when temperatures again become favourable, can germinate to form vegetative cells capable of reproduction. Some psychrophiles remain active at refrigerator temperatures, and some spores can even survive freezer temperatures.

Thus, low-temperature preservation cannot be expected to thoroughly destroy spoilage or pathogenic microorganisms in food. However, a reduction in the rate of microbial reproduction (along with a decrease in the number of cells) can be expected if correct time-temperature combinations are followed. The number of microorganisms killed, deactivated, or unaffected by low-temperature food preservation methods depends on the type and number of microbes present, the rate of cooling, the time temperature combinations, the characteristics of the food, and other variables. Low temperature food preservation is effective in many applications, particularly in controlling thermophiles and mesophiles. There are three kinds of low-temperature food preservation: chilled storage, refrigerated storage, and freezer storage.

Low temperatures preserve food products during their flow through the control points of a food service operation. They slow the growth of spoilage organisms and decrease the rate of chemical reactions and enzyme activity. The rate of microbial reproduction decreases as the temperature drops, and eventually stops altogether. Some organisms may survive the low temperatures and form spores which, when temperatures again become favourable, can germinate to form vegetative cells capable of reproduction. Some psychrophiles remain active at refrigerator temperatures, and some spores can even survive freezer temperatures.

Thus, low-temperature preservation cannot be expected to thoroughly destroy spoilage or pathogenic microorganisms in food. However, a reduction in the rate of microbial reproduction (along with a decrease in the number of cells) can be expected if correct time-temperature combinations are followed. The number of microorganisms killed, deactivated, or unaffected by low-temperature food preservation methods depends on the type and number of microbes present, the rate of cooling, the time temperature combinations, the characteristics of the food, and other variables. Low temperature food preservation is effective in many applications, particularly in controlling thermophiles and mesophiles.

There are three kinds of low-temperature food preservation:

1. chilled storage,
2. refrigerated storage, and
3. freezer storage.

Chilled storage: Temperatures for chilled storage are lower than room temperature but higher than those for refrigerated temperatures. A typical range for chilled storage is between 50 F (10°C) and 59°P (15°C). Some fruits and vegetables (potatoes and cucumbers, for example) should be stored in this range. Chilled storage may not be used for potentially hazardous foods.

Refrigerated storage: Temperatures for refrigerated storage range from 32°P (O°C) to 45F (7°C). Some jurisdictions specify 41F (5°C) as the highest refrigerated temperature; check your local regulations. Most food products that are classified as perishable are best stored at refrigerator temperatures. Storage at these temperatures slows the growth rate of spoilage organisms and most pathogenic bacteria (with the exception of some strains of Clostridium botulinum and certain psychrophiles). Enzymatic and chemical reactions are also significantly reduced at refrigerator temperatures.

Several factors affect the ability of refrigerator temperatures to control spoilage organisms. One factor is the relative humidity-the ratio of water vapour present in the air to the quantity of water vapour that would be present if the air were saturated at the same temperature. In other words, the relative humidity reports the amount of moisture in the air as a percentage. The relative humidity of a storage area affects microbial growth and, therefore, storage times. Excessive moisture encourages the growth of microorganisms. If the relative humidity is too low, food in storage loses moisture to the environment. Moisture loss in fresh fruits and vegetables is characterised by wilting, softening, shrinkage, and reduced weight.

Ventilation or air flow maintains a uniform level of relative humidity. Ventilation in storage areas also helps maintain an optimum storage environment by removing undesirable odours. In some cases, ventilation systems are used to alter the storage area atmosphere. The use of carbon dioxide gas or nitrogen gas makes it possible to maintain higher storage temperatures and relative humidities. It also prolongs the shelf life of food products. Such controlled-atmosphere storage methods are useful in maintaining the quality of fresh fruits and vegetables.

Freezer storage: Freezer storage temperatures are generally 0 F (-18°C) and below. As one would expect, these very low temperatures reduce the growth rate of microorganisms even further. But some spores can survive freezer storage temperatures. One advantage of freezing over refrigeration is that freezing also reduces the aw (water activity) of food products: when water is converted from liquid to solid form, microbes can no longer use it. Only high-quality food products should be selected for freezer storage because most food products lose quality after being frozen.

Any physical evidence of food spoilage or damage should be removed before freezing food products. All inedible parts of the food should also be removed. Fruit and vegetable products must be sorted, washed, and blanched before freezing. Blanching, the process of exposing the product to either steam or hot water for a short time sets the colour of green vegetables and renders enzymes inactive. The blanching process also destroys some microorganisms, forces trapped air out of the plant cells, and causes leafy vegetables to wilt, making them easier to pack.

Chemicals may be added to food products prior to freezing. Antioxidants are incorporated into some bakery products to prevent rancidity, a chemical change or decomposition in fats and oils, which produces a disagreeable taste or odor in foods. Ascorbic acid (vitamin C) is added to some fruits and vegetables to minimise browning during frozen storage.

Many people are surprised to learn that frozen fruits and vegetables may have a higher nutritive value than their "fresh" counterparts. Consider fresh grapefruit harvested in Florida and shipped to Michigan. The citrus fruit might take one or two days to reach the northern state. Once it is received by the food distributor in Michigan, it could be stored under refrigeration for a couple of weeks until a food service operation places an order. Upon delivery, it could be stored for as long as a week before it is actually used. Throughout this period, the fruit loses vitamin C. On the other hand, grapefruit to be commercially frozen is processed much more quickly, sometimes immediately after harvest. Therefore, the vitamin C content of frozen grapefruit is often higher than that of "fresh" grapefruit.

Quick freezing reduces the temperature of a product to -4 of (-20°C) in 30 minutes or less, while slow freezing takes 3 to 72 hours. Quick freezing is more desirable than slow freezing for a number of reasons. First, quick freezing better preserves product quality. Quick freezing causes small ice crystals to form within food, which minimises damage to the food's cell structure, thus preserving its flavour and texture. Second, when thawed, products that have been quick-frozen exhibit less drip loss than similar products that have been slow-frozen. Third, quick freezing slows enzymatic and microbial activity more promptly. However, the specialised equipment needed for quick freezing is seldom present in a food establishment, so slow-freezing methods are often used. In fact, most food service freezers are storage freezers designed to hold already-frozen products-not to freeze them.

A variety of quick-freezing methods are used for food products, depending on the individual characteristics of the product type. Immersion freezing entails dipping food products (such as fish fillets) directly into a low-temperature coolant. Liquid nitrogen, brine, or sugar solutions are used in this technique. Plate freezing is used for boxes and packages of food, such as 2 or 2 ½ pound (0.91 or 1.14 kg) boxes of frozen vegetables: each package is placed between two plates that have a low-temperature coolant passing through them. Blast freezing requires exposure of food to temperatures as low as 0F (-18°C) to -30°F (-34°C). This technique is used for freezing meats, fish, poultry, fruits, and vegetables.

Even when a food product is frozen and stored at freezer temperatures, several changes that adversely affect quality can still take place. Freezer burn is a dehydration that occurs when frozen products are not wrapped or packaged properly. This loss of moisture takes place on the surface of fruits, vegetables, meats, fish, and poultry. Unfortunately, freezer burn is irreversible. It is a form of food spoilage because it renders food products unusable. Furthermore, the texture, colour, odor, appearance, and taste of foods are slowly altered under freezer storage conditions.

Low-temperature preservation needs in food service operations have changed dramatically over the past several years. Operations that once relied heavily on dry storage areas for canned goods and frozen storage areas for frozen products have experienced a number of changes. The demand for fresh produce and fresh fish has created the need for more refrigerated storage space. Also, the move by some food distributors to minimise daily deliveries has led to bulk sale incentives and larger inventories of refrigerated items in food service operations.

Unfortunately, many older food service facilities were not designed with adequate refrigerated storage space for today's menu items. However, when replacement refrigeration equipment is purchased or when new facilities are constructed, many operators now install a single unit called a refrigerator-freezer or dual temperature unit. Thawing.

Frozen food products may be cooked directly from the frozen state or thawed prior to cooking. But frozen food thawing is potentially hazardous if food products are exposed to the temperature danger zone-the range of temperatures from 41°F (S°C) to 140°F (60°C). Remember, the TDZ may be different in your locality. The defrosting method selected should minimise contact with the TDZ. Never thaw frozen foods at room temperature. The risks are too great.

Recall that some frozen foods undergo a process known as slacking that allows the temperature of the food to gradually increase from -10°F (-23°C) to 2SOF (-4°C). Slacking is done in preparation for deep fat frying or to facilitate even heat penetration during the cooking of previously block-frozen food such as spinach.

Thawing under refrigeration at temperatures of 41°F (S°C) or less is recommended since it minimises contact with the TDZ. This method also minimises product quality loss and exposure to contamination. It works well for frozen fruit, poultry, fish, shellfish, and large cuts of meat. There is an added advantage to thawing under refrigeration: frozen food placed in a refrigerator to thaw will draw heat from the other refrigerated products. This heat exchange saves energy by reducing the amount of time the refrigerator's cooling equipment has to run. Today's food establishments are often designed with back-to-back walk-in freezer and refrigerator combinations. This design allows the (outer) refrigerator to serve as a buffer zone between the heat of the kitchen and the freezer, thus reducing the amount of cold air lost from the freezer.

Thawing under cold running water (70°F [21°C] or less) is also acceptable. Items thawed in this manner must be protected from water damage by being tightly wrapped or placed in watertight containers. This method works well with frozen fruit. Some jurisdictions do not recommend thawing potentially hazardous foods under cold running water. With some food products, defrosting as part of the cooking process can save time and still is safe. Small cuts of meat, poultry, fish, and frozen vegetables are usually defrosted and cooked simultaneously. Breaded vegetables, fish, and shellfish are actually better when they are cooked directly from the frozen state.

Microwave oven thawing may be used for some food products, although there are limitations. Microwave thawing is acceptable only when it is part of the cooking process or when it is followed immediately by cooking. Bread and rolls are toughened when heated in a microwave oven, and large pieces of meat may not fit into the chamber. It is important to remember that since foods are not pure water, they are not frozen at 32°F (0°C) as water is. Foods freeze and thaw at temperatures between 25°F (-4°C) and 32°F (D°C). Frozen foods have several opportunities to defrost during handling, transportation, and storing. If the food is thawed and then refrozen, large ice crystals will form and will reduce the quality.

Another low-temperature food preservation technique uses reduced oxygen packaging and is rapidly emerging due to technological advances. Sous vide (literally under vacuum) was invented by French chef George Pralus. The method consists of packaging food items into plastic bags or pouches, vacuum-sealing the pouches, and cooking the pouches of food while carefully controlling both moisture and temperature. The food is then immediately chilled to stop the cooking and stored refrigerated. The pouches may be reheated in hot water for service, or the fully cooked food may be served chilled.

Initially, the United States Food and Drug Administration (FDA) banned on-premises sous vide preparation in restaurants, citing the section of the 1976 Model Ordinance that refers to home-canned foods. The concern was due to the possibility of inadequate heat treatment, followed by the growth of Clostridium botulinum and the psychrophilic pathogens such as Listeria monocytogenes and Yersinia enterocolitica. Because of strict processing controls, sous vide preparation was only permitted in food processing plants and sold to food service operations.

High-Temperature Preservation

High temperatures are effective in food preservation because they control the growth of microorganisms. When most microbial cells are heated, they are either injured and deactivated or destroyed. The exceptions are thermophiles, which prefer higher temperatures, and other microorganisms, which have the ability to form heat - resistant spores. The heat stability of vegetative cells and spores varies considerably among species.

Several variables affect the survival rate of cells and spores exposed to high temperatures. First, the time-temperature relationship is critical to controlling the growth of microorganisms. With sufficiently high temperatures, the time required for microbial deactivation or destruction is reduced as the temperature is increased. Second, the initial colony size influences the rate of deactivation or destruction. Everything being equal, as the number of cells or spores initially presents increases, the amount of heat needed to accomplish deactivation or destruction also rises.

Finally, the composition of a food product also determines the effectiveness of high temperature food preservation. In general, carbohydrates, proteins, and fats in food protect some organisms from destruction by heat. When the aw is reduced, some microbes become more heat-resistant. A pH near 7.0 (neutral) also makes microorganisms more heat-resistant. Some food products may require added chemicals such as nitrites or preservatives to overcome microbial resistance to heat.

There are two methods of high-temperature food preservation:

1. pasteurisation
2. sterilisation.

Pasteurisation: Pasteurisation temperatures are used either to extend the shelf life of food by reducing spoilage organisms or to destroy all pathogenic microorganisms present in the food. Pasteurisation may be done in one of two ways. The holder process of pasteurisation involves heating the food product to 145°F (63°C) for 30 minutes. In the high temperature short time (HTST) method of pasteurisation, the product is heated to 161°F (72°C) for 15 seconds. Both techniques require the heated food to be immediately cooled to 50°F (l0°e) or less.

The most common example of pasteurised food is fluid milk. Either pasteurisation method can be used for milk and milk products, although the HTST process is preferred since it is so rapid. In either case, the time-temperature combination is sufficient to eliminate the possible presence of two pathogens:

1. Mycobacterium tuberculosis and
2. Coxiella burnetti.

These non-spore-forming pathogens cannot survive either pasteurisation method. The importance of the pasteurisation process is readily apparent when one considers that more than 17 billion gallons of milk are produced annually in the United States. In addition to milk, the government requires that ice cream mixes and liquid egg products (such as shelled whole eggs) be pasteurised. This process minimises the risk of Salmonella spp. microorganisms. Canned hams are also pasteurised. Pasteurisation eliminates pathogens, but since it does not destroy all microorganisms present in the food products, pasteurised foods must still be stored under refrigeration.

Sterilisation: Sterilisation destroys virtually all microorganisms and their spores. Once the food is batch-sterilised, or before it is individually sterilised, it must be stored in a hermetically sealed container, such as a can, glass bottle, or jar. With advances in food technology, flexible plastic containers can now be used for sterilised food products as well. Because the food is sterilised and hermetically sealed, it need not be refrigerated until the containers are opened.

The canning process is designed to achieve commercial sterilisation of food products. The process has improved greatly since Nicolas Appert did his pioneer work in canning in the late 1700s and early 1800s. The modern canning process begins with the arrival of the freshly harvested or slaughtered food. The food is cleaned and all inedible parts are removed.

Some vegetables are blanched prior to being placed in cans. The food is placed in washed cans, and brine (salt water) is added to vegetables. Fish products such as tuna may be packed in either brine or oil. A sugar-water solution is usually added to fruits during filling, although fruits packed in their own juices have gained popularity among consumers in recent years.

Once they are filled, the containers are evacuated; that is, a partial vacuum is created in the container. During the sealing stage, the lids are added and sealed to the body of the containers to form an airtight or hermetic seal. After the containers are sealed, they are heated to sterilisation temperatures for carefully controlled time periods.

A number of variables affect the amount of heat required for sterilisation. First, the size, shape, and material of the container affect the heat transfer rate. Smaller cans permit a faster heat transfer than larger cans or glass bottles. Second, the contents of the container have a tremendous effect on the heat transfer rate. Extremely viscous food products (for example, tomato paste) have a slower heat transfer rate than food products that are largely liquid (tomato puree). The pH of the food also influences the amount of heat necessary for sterilisation. In general, food products can be placed in one of three categories based on their pH:

1. *Low-acid foods (pH above 4.5)* include meats, fish, poultry, milk, spinach, asparagus, pumpkin, corn, and lima beans. Because of their low acid content, these products require a relatively severe heat treatment to guard against the growth of Clostridium botulinum. The sterilisation process is frequently used to achieve a desirable level of microbial destruction, while minimising the negative effects on the product's texture, taste, odor, colour, and appearance.
2. *Medium-acid foods (pH of 3.7 to 4.5)* include some tomatoes, pineapples, and pears. The acidity in this group of food products inhibits the growth of Clostridium botulinum. However, spoilage organisms can grow at this level of acidity, so the heat treatment must be severe enough to destroy these undesirable microbes.
3. *High-acid foods (pH below 3.7)* include sauerkraut and berries. Few pathogenic or spoilage organisms can survive in such high acidity. A relatively mild heat treatment is required for this group.

Heating for sterilisation usually takes place in a large container, which is pressurised according to the food product and its ability to withstand heat. Food products that are particularly sensitive to heat are processed using a variation of the normal canning process known as aseptic canning. This process involves the separate sterilisation of containers (using hydrogen peroxide) and contents, and uses more heat for substantially shorter periods of time than conventional canning. Once sterilised, the contents are placed into the containers and packed in a sterile environment. This process conserves nutrients, colour, taste, odor, and texture but is relatively expensive.

After the heating process is completed, the containers are cooled. The cooling process must be gradual to prevent cans from bending and bottles from cracking. Once they have cooled, the containers are labeled and placed in boxes or bottles for later shipment. Modern technology has made commercial canning a highly automated, continuous process.

Food Dehydration

Food dehydration may be the oldest method of food preservation. Primitive people probably discovered this method when they accidentally left food out in the sun. Dehydration is an effective method of preservation because it reduces the aw of food and thus inhibits microbial activity. There are four methods of drying food:

1. sun drying,
2. mechanical drying,
3. freeze-drying, and
4. drying during smoking.

Sun drying: This is effective in areas with low humidity and high temperatures. Fruits and vegetables have been dehydrated this way for centuries. Today, grapes, plums, currants, and apricots are dehydrated by this method.

Mechanical drying: This is the drying method of primary commercial importance. Food products are prepared for mechanical drying by trimming, washing, and removing the inedible parts. Then heat is applied, usually in combination with moving air. The three mechanical drying methods are spray drying, tunnel drying, and drum drying.

Spray drying is used for liquid foods. The liquid is sprayed continuously into the top of a drying chamber that may be several stories high. Hot air mixes with the falling food and evaporates the moisture. The result is a fine powder of dried food, which exits at the bottom of the chamber. Milk, tea, eggs, coffee, and fruit purees are spray dried.

Tunnel drying uses a conveyor belt to move the food products into and out of a drying chamber. Like spray drying, tunnel drying is a continuous process. Once in the chamber, the food is exposed to blasts of hot air that evaporate moisture. Tunnel drying is used for vegetables, fruits, nuts, confectionery products, and breakfast cereals.

Drum drying uses a large rotating drum heated from within by steam. Liquid food is applied to the drum in a thin film as it rotates. A scraper is used to remove the dried food from the drum in this continuous process. Potatoes, breakfast cereals, infant foods, soups, and sauces are dried using this mechanical process.

Freeze-drying: This technique uses a process known as sublimation-the direct conversion of solid water (ice) to water vapour without the usual intermediate step of melting into a liquid. To freeze-dry a product, the product must first be frozen. Sublimation takes place in a drying chamber where a vacuum and a small amount of heat are applied. This process results in a dried product that is porous and easy to rehydrate. The food product suffers minimal damage because only a small amount of heat is required for this process. However, freeze-drying is relatively expensive. Freeze-drying has been used for meat, fish, shellfish, poultry, vegetables, fruits, and coffee.

Chemical Food Preservation

Several chemical food additives have been approved by the Food and Drug Administration for, food preservation applications. These chemical preservatives inhibit the activity of selected pathogens and spoilage organisms. The FDA strictly monitors the use of chemical preservatives. The categories of chemical preservatives are nitrites and nitrates, sugar and salt, sulfur dioxides and sulfites, ethylene and propylene oxides, alcohol, organic acids and their salts, and spices and other condiments.

Nitrites, nitrates, and their salts are used in the preservation of meat products. They inhibit the activity of Clostridium botulinum, give cured meats their typical colour, and contribute to flavour. Nitrites and nitrates are added to bacon, lunch meats, ham, and other cured meats. Recently, the USDA approved a reduction in the amount of nitrite preservatives added to bacon, from 120 parts per million (ppm) to 100 ppm. Note that milligrams/liter (mg/L) is the metric equivalent.

An alternative approved method is to use lactic acid starter cultures and sugar in a curing solution, with 40 mg/L to 80 mg/L of sodium nitrite. This will result in savings for food service operations while maintaining safety. Sugar and salt bind water and lower a food product's aw. Salt is used in brines in which canned fish, meats, and vegetables are packed, and enhances their flavour. Sugar is found in the syrups in which canned fruits are packed; it also contributes to their flavour. Salt and sugar are added to a wide variety of processed foods as preservatives. Sulfiting agents (sulfur dioxide, sodium sulfite, sodium and potassium bisulfite, and sodium and potassium metabisulfite) have been used to retard oxidative or enzymatic browning of fruits and vegetables, to inhibit "black spot" on shrimp, and to control gray mold on table grapes. Since sulfites bind to food constituents, they remain in or on food in spite of washing. Cooking, particularly the high heat of frying reduces sulfite residues but does not eliminate them.

The FDA has banned the use of sulfites in raw fruits and vegetables intended to be served or sold raw. The FDA has also proposed to ban sulfites in fresh potato products and limit sulfite levels in beer, wine, baked goods, tea, and fruit juices. Sulfites have been known to cause severe reactions and even death in asthmatics. The FDA has reminded food service operators that the federal rules do not replace state and local rules. Some countries have banned the application of sulfites in food establishments. It is a good idea to be certain that your food and beverage operation complies with regulations issued by local health authorities.

Ethylene and propylene oxides are used to sterilise containers in which food is packaged. For example, wine bottles and juice packages are sterilised with these oxides before the beverages are added.

Ethanol (ethyl alcohol), which functions as a preservative, is produced by fermentation in wine, beer, and spirits. The natural flavourings in these beverages are dissolved in the ethanol. Ethanol is also the main flavour carrier in extracts used for cooking (for example, almond and vanilla extracts).

Organic acids and their salts are sometimes added to food products as preservatives. Salts are formed when organic acids and metals (for example, sodium, calcium, and potassium) are combined. However, in some foods, these acids and salts form naturally during normal fermentation. Benzoates are salts derived from benzoic acid and are added to carbonated beverages, pickled vegetables, fruit jams and jellies, and margarine. Propionates are salts made from propionic acid. They control mold growth in baked products and cheeses. Sorbates, derived from sorbic acid, inhibit mold and yeast activity. Sorbates are added to cheeses, beverages, fruits, margarine, pickled vegetables, and jams and jellies.

Acetates are derivatives of acetic acid, better known as vinegar. Acetates are used in pickled vegetables, condiments, pickled sausages, and mayonnaise. Ascorbic acid, erythorbic acid, citric acid, sodium ascorbate, and sodium citrate are used to maintain the colour and overall appearance of fresh pork.

One major advance in chemical food preservation is the use of organic acids to lower the pH of food products. Certain operations (commissaries and chain operations, for example) can afford the equipment, technology, and monitoring systems to use pH adjustments as a complement to correct time-temperature combinations. Standard recipes can be adjusted by the addition of organic acids and high-acid food ingredients to produce a product with a lower pH. While pH adjustments are currently not suitable for every food item or operation, this method of preservation has the potential for widespread application in the future.

Spices and other condiments constitute the last class of chemical preservatives. Not all spices and condiments have the effect of inhibiting bacterial activity in food products, but some have been valued for centuries as flavour enhancers and preservatives. Cinnamon and cloves have anti-microbial properties. Condiments that contain vinegar also discourage the growth of pathogens and spoilage organisms.

Mayonnaise, which is often wrongly blamed for foodborne illness outbreaks traced to salads, kills

Staphylococcus aureus, Escherichia coli, and Salmonella spp. However, high protein foods (such as meat, poultry, fish, and eggs), when added to mayonnaise, raise the product's pH and increase the likelihood of microbial growth. Holding salads in the temperature danger zone (41 ° to 1400P [5° to 60°C]) compounds the risks.

Radiation in Food Preservation

The use of radiation in food preservation is presently limited, although further research may reveal new applications. This method of preservation, called irradiation, involves exposing food to ultraviolet light, gamma rays, or X rays to destroy harmful organisms. Ultraviolet light acts only on the surface of food products. In the past, it was used in the aging (tenderisation) of meats at relatively high temperatures. Ultraviolet light is now used to reduce bacterial activity on the surface of fruitcakes before they are wrapped.

Gamma rays are produced by radioactive elements such as cobalt. These short length waves disrupt cell components and kill harmful microorganisms and insects. They can be used to sterilise or pasteurise food products such as meat and poultry. In some instances, they are used to reduce insect infestation in newly harvested grains. Low doses of gamma rays add little heat to food while allowing flavours to remain intact and extending shelf life significantly. High doses of gamma rays negatively alter the colour, odor, taste, and appearance of foods.

Current research and development of low dosage gamma radiation may result in a preservation technique that will not significantly alter either the appearance or taste of food. Fruits, vegetables, fish, and poultry are some of the products that could be preserved by low dosage gamma radiation in the future. X rays are essentially the same as gamma rays.

Food irradiation can help extend shelf life by keeping grains from sprouting, deactivating molds, and killing spoilage bacteria. It can also make food safer. At low to medium doses, radiation kills Salmonella spp. and other pathogens, including the parasite Trichinella spiralis.

Consumer concerns have been raised that irradiation will produce new chemical compounds in foods. However, researchers have concluded that the changes in food resulting from irradiation are too small to affect the safety of the food product. Irradiated foods contain chemicals identical to those found in baked or broiled foods, and contain fewer altered chemicals than barbecued steak. Consumers are not exposed to radiation by eating irradiated food, since the process of irradiation is low in intensity and the energy passes through the food leaving no radioactivity.

One scientist has said that consumers run no more risk of being exposed to radiation from irradiated food than they do from a briefcase that has been X-rayed by a machine at an airport. Nevertheless, consumers and health groups concerned with the effects of food irradiation petitioned the FDA to require warnings on menus and on the doors of restaurants offering irradiated foods for sale. The groups asked the FDA to require the word "picowaved" and the international symbol for food irradiation.

In a survey conducted by the Food Marketing Institute (FMI), over 70% of the respondents characterised irradiated foods as a hazard. Fewer than 30% of the respondents indicated that they had even heard of food irradiation two years earlier. The FDA has ruled that even though foods preserved through irradiation must be labeled to show this fact at both the wholesale and retail levels, "multiple-ingredient foods" such as restaurant meals are exempt from this requirement. The FDA's ruling stated that the effects of radiation on individual ingredients would likely have no significant effect on the final product. Further changes can be expected as technology improves and consumer groups become more active and vocal.

One additional method of preserving foods is known as pulsed-power. This method uses tens of thousands of volts of electricity in bursts as brief as millionths of a second to kill bacteria and extend shelf life. Other technological advances may permit the use of pulsed electromagnetic fields to do the same thing.

Having explored the causes of food spoilage and the methods of commercial preservation, we can now consider specific recommendations for preserving various types of food. The recommendations which follow should be valuable to food service and lodging businesses, considering the large sums of money they spend on food products. These recommendations can help eliminate the risk of serving spoiled food products to guests.

Preservation Methods for Various Types of Foods

This section covers the characteristics, spoilage potential, and preservation methods for each group of food products. The two main categories are foods from animal sources and foods from plant sources, although fats and oils overlap these categories somewhat. Within each main category, some foods have their own unique preservation methods.

Preservation of Non-vegetables

Non-vegetable foods items include meat, poultry, fish and shellfish, eggs, dairy products, and fats. These foods represent a large portion of the food dollars spent by the average food service operation, so their preservation is important.

Meat

Meat is generally defined as the flesh of any animal used for food. For purposes of this discussion, meat includes beef, lamb, veal, and pork. Meat and meat products are considered potentially hazardous foods. Several pathogenic bacteria have been detected in fresh meat products. Among the most prominent are Staphylococcus aureus, Salmonella spp., Clostridium perfringens, Listeria monocytogenes, Yersinia enterocolitica, Campylobacter jejuni, and the parasite Trichinella spiral is. Spoilage organisms have also been detected in fresh meat products.

Generally, the normal muscle tissue of healthy living animals does not harbour pathogenic microorganisms. However, spoilage organisms and pathogens can invade the muscle tissue from the animal's intestinal tract when the animal is slaughtered. The extent of the invasion depends on the following factors:

— The microbial content of the animal's intestines

— The physiological condition of the animal before slaughter

— The method of slaughter

— The method of carcass cooling

The microbial content of the animal's intestines probably exerts the greatest influence over potential contamination. For this reason, meat animals are usually starved for 24 hours before they are slaughtered.

The animal's physiological condition determines its internal body chemistry to some extent. Normally, after an animal is slaughtered, its muscles become stiff-a condition known as rigor mortis. Rigor mortis takes place in meat animals about 6 to 12 hours after slaughter, depending on the carcass size. As rigor mortis sets in, a chemical reaction called anaerobic glycolysis takes place, during which glycogen (a chemical form of energy stored in muscle tissue) is converted to lactic acid. Calm, rested animals have more glycogen in their muscle tissues; thus, the production of lactic acid after slaughter causes a dramatic pH drop (from 7.0 to 5.6). An animal that is excited or fatigued before slaughtering will have used up its stored glycogen, and thus less lactic acid will be produced and the pH drop will not be as dramatic. The result is dark cutting meat, which is less tender and more susceptible to microbial attack.

The method of slaughter should be quick and efficient. Besides being more humane, quick slaughtering can accomplish the objective of rapid bleeding in a relatively sanitary environment. The method of carcass cooling is also important to meat preservation. Carcasses must be cooled quickly to reduce contact with the temperature danger zone. Additional microorganisms might be introduced after an animal is slaughtered. Contaminants might enter the meat tissue from the animal's hide when it is skinned.

When meat products are cut up or boned, further contamination might be introduced through knives and cutting surfaces. Ground (comminuted) meats and finely chopped meats are most susceptible to contamination because of their large surface areas, due to a reduction in size by chopping, flaking, grinding, or mincing, and the additional handling they receive. Nevertheless, most meat contamination comes from the penetration of pathogens from the intestinal tract of the animal.

The survival and growth of microorganisms in meat are influenced by the kinds of organisms present, the physical and chemical characteristics of the meat, the storage temperature, and the amount of available oxygen. Besides being subject to contamination with pathogens, which has already been discussed, meats are susceptible to two broad types of spoilage: anaerobic and aerobic.

Anaerobic spoilage of meat tissue takes place under conditions with a limited amount of oxygen. Putrefaction is a bacterial splitting of meat proteins, resulting in the formation of foul odours. Pseudomonas spp. is the bacteria responsible for this type of spoilage. Souring is a form of anaerobic spoilage caused by the production of acids. This process results in a sour odor and taste in meats.

Aerobic spoilage of meat tissue is likelier to occur since fresh meat is rarely stored in an oxygen-free environment. Bacteria are responsible for the greatest amount of aerobic meat spoilage. Some bacteria form slimy capsules and surface slime on meat. Other bacteria change the colour of meat to gray, green, and shades of brown. Still others cause fat rancidity in meats. Finally, surface colours on meat can be changed to red, green, blue, or yellow by bacteria that produce pigments.

Molds are aerobic organisms that cause fuzziness or stickiness on meats. Colour changes (green, black, and white) are caused by molds. Other molds can decompose fats and proteins in meats because they have enzymes that accelerate the breakdown. This results in an unacceptable odor, colour, taste, texture, and appearance. The genus of molds called Penicillium is often responsible for meat spoilage.

Food preservation methods for meat products are designed to prevent the activity of pathogenic and spoilage microorganisms. Meat products may be rendered commercially sterile by the canning process. Meat products may also be pasteurised and then stored under refrigeration. Low-temperature preservation is the commonest method of preserving fresh meats. Freezing and refrigerating are preferable to canning in that they do not significantly alter the taste and texture of meat. However, some psychrophilic spoilage organisms (Pseudomonas spp.) can grow on meats stored at refrigerator temperatures. Whenever meat products are chilled or frozen, they should be carefully wrapped to minimise contamination and dehydration.

Some meat products are preserved by drying. This was a common practice among the pioneers who settled the western part of the United States: they made jerky by cutting meat into strips and drying it in the sun. Modern-day adventurers who backpack in the wilderness often take foil-packaged freeze-dried meat products, which are easy to carry and prepare. Freeze dried meat products are shelf stable as long as they are stored properly and their packages are not opened. Other dried meat products are often cured and/or smoked. Curing is the addition of common table salt, sugar, nitrites, or nitrates to meats. Smoking provides additional flavour to crude meats and helps to tenderise beef and pork products. Meat can also be dried by smoking alone.

The USDA has developed a simple, fast, and inexpensive test to measure potential spoilage in ground beef. The test measures lactic acid; high levels of this organic acid indicate that the beef will spoil quickly and develop a sour odor. The test is being used by food service distributors and may find its way into food service operations.

An increasing number of food service operations are offering "exotic meats" on their menus. Wild game, for example, may be served in a food service operation provided the food products have been obtained from an approved and safe source. Since these food products are not usually raised commercially, extra caution is necessary.

Poultry

This category includes chicken, turkey, duck, goose, and game birds. Like meats, poultry products are classified as potentially hazardous foods. Pathogenic and spoilage organisms prefer poultry products because they have a favourable pH, high moisture content, and high nitrogen content. The intestinal tract and skin of poultry may contain a variety of pathogenic bacteria, including Staphylococcus aureus, Salmonella spp., and Escherichia coli. Other pathogens that have been associated with poultry products include Clostridium perfringens, Listeria monocytogenes, and Campylobacter jejuni.

The frequent identification of poultry products with cases of human salmonellosis makes it especially important to properly handle and preserve poultry products. Spoilage is apparent when poultry is sticky, slimy, and has an objectionable odor. Generally, two types of spoilage affect poultry products. Enzymes, present within the poultry cell, can cause chemical changes and deterioration.

Fortunately, enzymatic changes are significantly slowed by refrigeration or freezing. Bacteria are responsible for even more poultry spoilage. Bacterial spoilage is usually traceable to the Pseudomonas and Flavobacterium genera. As with meat, most spoilage bacteria come from the live animal's skin and intestinal tract. Bacteria reproduce on the skin of slaughtered birds, in the cavity of whole carcasses, and on any cut tissue. Slowly, these spoilage organisms penetrate into the poultry tissue. Molds also accelerate the spoilage of poultry products.

Many precautionary measures are taken to properly process poultry products. After the birds are slaughtered, the carcasses are washed with chlorinated water to kill germs. Then the carcasses are immediately chilled by cold air, ice, or iced water. The cold air method is preferred because it rapidly brings the temperature down to 32°F (O°C) and does not add extra moisture to the carcass. If the poultry is cut up, additional steps must be taken to ensure that contamination is not added.

Low-temperature preservation is frequently used for poultry products. Poultry products can be refrigerated or frozen successfully if they are carefully wrapped to minimise dehydration, contamination, and quality deterioration. Rapid freezing is desirable for the reasons previously discussed.

Poultry products may also be preserved with the addition of heat. Poultry may be canned whole, in pieces, or completely boned. Some canned poultry products have a chemical preservative added. Organic acids, such as acetic acid, lengthen the shelf life of poultry products by lowering the pH. Some turkey products are cured; others are cured and then smoked.

Fish

Consumption of fish is on the rise in the United States. Fish products may be subdivided into a number of categories, the most common being finfish and shellfish. Finfish come from freshwater lakes and rivers and from the ocean. Finfish can be classified as either fatty or lean. Fatty finfish include bluefish, bonito, mackerel, pompano, salmon, shark, smelt, swordfish, trout, tuna, and whitefish. Other species of finfish are generally classified as lean. Bass, cod, flounder, grouper, haddock, halibut, monkfish, ocean perch, snapper, sole, tilefish, turbot, and whiting fall into this category. Shellfish are also considered lean. Shellfish are classified as crustaceans, which include crab, lobster, and shrimp, or mollusks, which include abalone, clams, octopus, oysters, scallops, snails, and squid.

Finfish and shellfish have less connective tissue and a relatively high moisture content compared with meat and poultry. Therefore, finfish and shellfish are more susceptible than meats and poultry to enzymatic autolysis and microbial spoilage. Unlike meat and poultry processors, fish processors have no mandatory government inspections for quality or wholesomeness. However, there is increasing pressure to move toward mandatory government inspections because of the number of foodborne illness outbreaks associated with fish.

The industry is fragmented; East Coast fish are primarily harvested wild, while West Coast fish are usually farmed. Inspections are currently made at the supplier's discretion and cost. Fish inspection is further complicated by the absence of any safe sensory method for differentiating between toxic and nontoxic seafood. It is therefore very important for food service operators to get to know their fish suppliers and be assured that they are safe sources.

One of the trends in the production of fish and shellfish is cultivation, or aquaculture. After starting with trout farming, processors are now commercially raising catfish, clams, shrimp, oysters, mussels, crayfish, striped bass, and salmon. Research is ongoing in the aquaculture of lobsters, scallops, redfish, and sturgeon.

Fish cultivation provides readily renewable supplies, and the size, flavour, and nutrients can be tailored to market needs. In addition, the freedom from contact with pollutants and pathogenic organisms in the natural habitat is a major advantage. Aquaculture, along with more rigorous inspection procedures, will go a long way toward reducing the potential hazards of serving these products.

Contamination of fish can come from the natural slime present on the skin of fish. Most of this natural coating is harmless, but if the fish are taken from contaminated waters, their slime covering may be expected to contain contaminants. Typical pathogens on the skin of fish are Vibrio parahaemolyticus, Clostridium botulinum, Salmonella spp., and the virus of infectious hepatitis. Further contamination can be introduced during processing and handling. The intestinal tract of fish could contain pathogens of the genera Escherichia, Clostridium, and Bacillus.

Other pathogens that could be associated with fish are Staphylococcus aureus, the Norwalk virus, and the parasites Diphyllobothrium latum (freshwater fish) and Anisakis spp. (cod and herring). Spoilage organisms responsible for an ammonia like odour are Pseudomonas spp. and Proteus spp., while Acinetobacter spp. and Aeromonas spp. produce unpleasant fruity or sweet odours in spoiled fish. During receiving of fish or shellfish, a trained representative of the food service operation should check product temperature, condition of the cases the products are received in, freshness, wholesomeness, and integrity. These inspections should be completed before storing the products.

The products should be well iced or solidly frozen when received. Use a probe thermometer to determine product temperature, which should then be checked against the following temperature guidelines:

— 32° to 38°F (0° to 3°C) for fresh fish
— 0° to 10°F (-18° to -12°C) for frozen fish
— 41°F (S°C) or less for live mollusks
— 40°F (4°C) for live crabs and lobsters
— 38°F (3°C) or less for vacuum-packed, modified atmosphere-packed, and pasteurised products Any damaged cases should be opened, and any moisture or signs of dried moisture should be investigated.

Dairy Products

These products constitute the fifth category of foods from animal sources. This large category encompasses milk, cream, butter, cheese, frozen deserts, and fermented milk products. Most of these products begin with cows milk.

The milk of healthy cows contains few pathogens or spoilage organisms. However, contamination has been traced to equipment and handlers. Equipment may harbour Staphylococcus aureus and Salmonella spp. organisms. Other pathogens responsible for foodborne outbreaks with dairy products include Listeria monocytogenes, Campylobacter jejuni, and Yersinia enterocolitica. Because milk and milk products are highly perishable, they are classified as potentially hazardous foods.

Dairy products may spoil in a variety of ways. Fresh milk may sour by the action of Streptococcus lactis, Lactobacillus bulgaricus, or Lactobacillus thermophilus, depending on its temperature. While this souring is undesirable in milk and most other dairy products, it adds to the characteristic flavour of yogurt. When Bacillus, Clostridium, and Pseudomonas organisms are present in milk, a protein breakdown results. Other organisms are responsible for the rancidity of milk fat, flavour changes, and colour changes in milk. Dairy products are primarily preserved by pasteurisation, because the fresh milk used to make them is pasteurised.

Fresh milk is potentially hazardous and must be stored under exact time-temperature combinations. In the United States, fresh whole milk is usually homogenised, although this does not contribute to its preservation. Homogenisation is a process that uses pressure to force milk through tiny openings. This breaks up the fat globules present in whole milk so that they are permanently suspended in the whey (liquid portion of the milk). There the fat globules cannot recombine and rise to the top as cream. Before the process of homogenisation was widely used, consumers had to vigorously shake bottles of unhomogenised milk to distribute the milk fat-which recombined quickly. Many people prefer to drink low fat or skim milk; these products have some of the fat skimmed off before homogenisation. In addition to being pasteurised, condensed milk and evaporated milk are canned, so they last much longer than fresh milk. Few spoilage problems arise as long as their containers have been properly sealed and heat processed. The high sugar content of condensed milk also helps to preserve it.

Dried milk is made by heating milk and then spray-drying it. The combination of heat and drying usually results in low bacterial counts. Dried milk is relatively safe as long as it is properly stored to prevent the addition of moisture. Ice cream is generally free of bacteria. It benefits from the combination of pasteurisation and freezer temperatures, which kill most organisms and prevent the reproduction of survivors.

Butter is made from pasteurised cream. Once butter is produced, it is held at freezer temperatures. Butter containing salt is more inhibiting to bacteria than salt-free butter. The low moisture content of butter provides favourable conditions for mold growth. Cheese is manufactured from pasteurised milk. Some cheeses, such as Romano and Parmesan, are so low in moisture that they may not support the normal growth of bacteria. However, molds frequently attack cheeses. Cheese may be salted or smoked during processing.

Fats and oils

Fats and oils constitute an important food category because they are part of a wide variety of food products, including cookies, crackers, butter, cheese, breakfast cereals, salad dressings, milk, nuts, snack foods, meats, poultry, some fish, and some fruits and vegetables. Fats and oils in their pure form may be differentiated in three ways. Fats come from animal sources, are solid at room temperature, and are usually saturated. Oils are generally from plant sources, are liquid at room temperature, and are unsaturated.

Saturated fats contain the maximum amount of hydrogen in the molecule and are therefore less susceptible to breakdown than unsaturated oils.

Foods containing fats and oils can undergo three types of breakdown reactions: autoxidation, hydrolytic rancidity, and flavour reversion. Autoxidation is a form of oxidative rancidity caused by the exposure of the fat or oil to oxygen. The reaction is accelerated by the presence of heat, metals, salt, and light. Unsaturated oils are more susceptible to autoxidation than saturated fats. Oxidative rancidity gives off-odours and Flavours to food products. It is controlled by the addition of antioxidants such as BHA (butylated hydroxyanisole) and BHT (butylated hydroxy toluene). BHA and BHT are added to many bakery products to control autoxidation.

Hydrolytic rancidity is responsible for flavour, odour, and taste changes in butter and products containing milk fat. It is caused by an enzyme called lipase. Lipase breaks down milk fat into its components. Since the fatty acids in milk fat are saturated, they possess a noticeable odor at room temperature. This reaction is controlled by heating the milk fat to destroy the lipase enzyme.

Flavour reversion is another form of oxidative rancidity. It occurs in vegetable oils that are highly unsaturated and contain linolenic acid, a polyunsaturated fatty acid. The result of flavour reversion is an unacceptable beany, fishy, or paint-like odor. Flavour reversion is controlled by a process known as partial hydrogenation. Hydrogen gas is added so that the polyunsaturated linolenic fatty acid becomes saturated and the problem is eliminated. Soybean oils used in the manufacture of salad dressings are partially hydrogenated to control flavour reversion, as are other oils found in many processed foods. Fats and oils generally contain few, if any, pathogenic organisms.

The reasons for the proper preservation of foods obtained from animal sources are obvious. First, proper preservation controls pathogenic microorganisms, which could cause a foodborne disease outbreak. Thus, it contributes to the operation's sanitation risk management programme. Second, effective control of spoilage reduces food waste. Because foods from animal sources constitute the majority of purchases made by most food establishments, proper preservation of these products is essential to any operation's cost control programme. Finally, proper storage of foods preserves their desirable qualities and thus contributes to overall guest satisfaction.

Preservation of Foods from Plant Sources

Foods from plant sources have increased in popularity over the last several years; per capita consumption is up by nearly 30% since 1970.5 Fresh vegetables are preferred to frozen and canned by almost 2 to 1.6 In keeping with the trends toward physical fitness, weight consciousness, and nutritious, high-fiber diets, food service guests are demanding more fruits, vegetables, grains, cereals, and nuts.

Fresh Fruits and Vegetables

These products generally continue respiring (living) after they are harvested. As they pass through the distribution channels, their respiration is counteracted by autolysis and microbial spoilage. The rate of enzymatic autolysis in fruits and vegetables varies directly with the temperature. Autolysis is substantially reduced when temperatures are decreased.

A number of microorganisms may be present on the exteriors of fresh fruits and vegetables. The microbes include Pseudomonas spp., Shigella spp., Bacillus spp., Streptococcus faecalis, Staphylococcus aureus, Clostridium botulinum, and a variety of molds. Most of these are spoilage organisms, although a few are pathogenic to humans. Bacteria, are responsible for several types of vegetable spoilage. Psuedomonas spp. cause a mushy, soft, malodorous spoilage called soft rot. Other bacteria cause vegetables to rot and develop sour odours. Botrytis cinerea is a mold which causes gray rot on vegetables. Other molds can cause soft rot, black rot, and sour rot.

Most fruit spoilage is the result of mold growth. Molds may produce gray, green, blue, and white pigments on fruit. For example, Botrytis cinerea causes a gray rot, while Penicillium spp. are responsible for a blue-coloured rot. The activity of molds can also cause softening, souring, and the development of bitter flavours in fresh fruits. Fresh fruits and vegetables acquire their microbial populations from the water and the soil as they grow.

Since plants consist largely of moisture and carbohydrates, organisms, which prefer these nutrient sources, are most frequently found on fruits and vegetables. Surface washing reduces the exterior microbial population. Fresh fruits and vegetables are preserved by the use of low temperatures. When they are harvested, their temperature is immediately dropped for preservation purposes. Many fruits and vegetables can be frozen. Others are refrigerated as they move to fresh produce markets. However, some fruits (such as bananas) are susceptible to chill shock and must be stored at higher temperatures.

The year-round availability of fruits and vegetables throughout the United States is largely due to freezing and canning. Of course, some canned foods still spoil due to can corrosion, leakage, or insufficient heating during the canning process. Three types of canned food spoilage are flat sour spoilage, thermophilic gas spoilage, and carbon dioxide gas spoilage.

Flat sour spoilage of canned foods is caused by the anaerobic growth of heat resistant, spore-forming bacteria. Bacillus coagulans is responsible for this kind of spoilage in tomatoes and tomato juice. These organisms change the flavour (but not the appearance) of canned foods.

Thermophilic gas spoilage is also caused by heat-resistant microbes that form spores. However, when these microorganisms survive the heating process (due to insufficient timetemperature combinations), they produce gas. Examples are Clostridium sporogenes, Clostridium putrefaciens, and Clostridium thermosaccharolyticum. These organisms cause food cans to swell and become distorted. A "flipper" is a can with flat ends that bulge when the can is warm. A "springer" is a can with moderate bulges on both top and bottom.

A "soft swell" is similar to a springer; however, the bulges can be pushed back with finger pressure. A "hard swell" has bulges at both ends, which cannot be pushed back with finger pressure. In general, if the top and the bottom of a can are flat, it is a safe product. Carbon dioxide gas spoilage occurs when non-spore-forming bacteria enter the product after processing. These spoilage organisms get into the can through faulty seals or leaks. For example, Micrococcus spp. and Streptococcus thermophilus can make the contents of a can frothy and slimy. Carbon dioxide gas spoilage produces flippers, springers, soft swells, and hard swells. Of course, there is always the possibility that the deadly toxin of the pathogen Clostridium botulinum may be present in a swollen can. If you ever observe any abnormal conditions in canned products, throw them out. Do not take a chance with your own life or the lives of your guests and staff members.

Canned foods, with the exception of ethnic products and boxed fruit juices, are losing popularity in the United States. This is due largely to the increasing popularity of fresh fruits and vegetables. In addition to, freezing and canning, drying is used to preserve some fruits and vegetables. This process destroys molds and yeasts, as well as non-spore-forming bacteria. Freeze-drying is very effective with fruits and vegetables. Regardless of how fruits and vegetables are preserved, care must be taken to avoid introducing pathogenic and spoilage organisms during processing and handling.

With advances in technology, hydroponics might one-day help meet the food service industry's demand for fresh vegetables, fruits, and herbs. Hydroponics is the growing of fresh produce in a nutrient-enriched water solution. No soil is used, and nutrient levels are controlled by computer. A major advantage of this method is that it produces cleaner, less contaminated products. Even though it is relatively expensive at this time, hydroponics might be the wave of the future.

Cereals, Grains, and Flours

These products are various forms of wheat, oats, rice, barley, corn, rye, and chicory plants. They can be grouped together because they have similar contamination problems. The exterior of these products can be contaminated by soil, insects, and equipment. Bacillus cereus is an organism frequently found on cereal grains. Most microbial contamination is removed from grains during milling; thus flours are relatively free of pathogens and spoilage organisms. However, if the moisture content of flour is raised, certain bacteria can cause a fermentation, which results in spoilage. Molds frequently attack baked products made from flours.

Among the most familiar spoiled foods in this category are bakery products, which exhibit Rhizopus nigricans (a black mold) or Penicillium expansum (a green mold). Mold growth can be controlled in baked products by fast cooling, followed by prompt wrapping. The addition of chemicals to doughs and batters prior to baking also inhibits mold activity.

The formation of rope in bakery products is characterised by an odor of ripe melons, yellow crumb colour, sticky crumbs, and a slimy, thread-like material evident when the product is sliced. Rope is caused by a spore-forming group of Bacillus organisms. It is controlled by the addition of acid prior to baking fast cooling and freezing. Spices. Spices are normally not prone to spoilage, although they may have molds present.

Some spices exhibit bacterial spoilage if their water content is excessively increased. Nuts. Nuts do not normally spoil by the action of bacteria because their moisture content is too low and their fat content too high. They are susceptible to rancidity reactions, however. Molds can also cause some problems if the water content of the nuts is raised. Aspergillus flavus molds produce aflatoxins in peanuts.

Carbonated beverages

These products generally do not spoil if stored properly. The trapped carbon dioxide gas lowers the pH, and added acids inhibit microbial activity. Because yeasts can spoil carbonated beverages containing sugar, beverage canners and bottlers carefully control the yeast content of their products. Beer should be stored where it is not exposed to heat or light.

Most bottled and canned beer is pasteurised and, if stored below 70°F (21°C), will not spoil if used within 90 to 120 days of packaging. Keg beer is more delicate since it is usually not pasteurised. Table wine may be attacked by yeasts and bacteria; the result is the formation of acetic acid. Alcoholic spirits and liqueurs contain so much alcohol they are virtually free from all forms of spoilage.

6

Room Cleaning

Every guest expects a clean room. In fact, it is a hotel owner's requirement by state law to provide a clean room. Guest room decor may be old or new, contemporary or traditional, bright or subdued, but it must be clean and comfortable.

The comfortable part is the beds. Regardless of the number of chairs, guests will sit on the edge of the bed, thus requiring the turning and flipping of mattresses on a regular basis. Most chains require that this be done four times a year. Also, be sure to rotate the box springs once a year. These simple procedures will:

1. Extend the life of your bedding, saving you money.
2. Provide your guests with a more comfortable bed, and thus increase your repeat business, making you money.

How often do you clean the carpets? Possibly only when required by an accident or according to your general cleaning schedule. An owner once stated that the room carpets were fine, as he had the same carpet in his apartment. However, after he was requested to walk in guest rooms with clean white socks, he had visible evidence of the dirt in the carpets, validating guest complaints. In high-occupancy hotels, try to clean a room carpet every six weeks.

The "sanitized" paper band placed on commodes is a waste of time and money. That is why the most noted chains do not require them. What they do require is a sparkling, shining clean commode, and that is accomplished only by using bowl cleaner and a commode brush. Clean the bathtub, shine the chrome, and don't forget the paper trash under the bed and behind the dresser.

Restroom Cleaning

Vapour Cleaning

These restroom cleaning systems are becoming increasingly popular. The systems use no chemicals. Instead, they use a tank that superheats the water, and operators spray the resulting steam onto the dirty areas with a special wand that features an applicator to which cleaning towels might be attached. The operator wipes all surfaces with the superheated vapor, changing the cloth as it becomes soiled. The units also have special heads that allow for crevice cleaning.

In addition to using these units for cleaning restrooms, cleaning crews also can use them for cleaning kitchens because the steam easily breaks down the grease. Also, when using the wand and towel attachment, the units might be effective in cleaning dirt off walls.

Manufacturers of some of these systems claim that the units require no chemicals, but housekeeping managers should familiarize themselves with the claims and the infection-control needs of their facility. Also, operators need to be aware that the vapor is hot and that handles of some wands might become hot. As a result, they will need to wear appropriate personal protective equipment.

Several manufacturers now market restroom cleaning kits that might include a cleaning cart, a bucket and a series of extension handles with associated specialized mop heads and attachments. The cart has space for storing cleaning supplies and paper products. Increasingly, crews are replacing old cotton-string mops with microfiber flat mops that are easier to use, lighter and enable aggressive cleaning of the surface.

The restroom cleaning kits give the person cleaning restrooms all of the necessary products they might need on the job site. Some advocates of microfiber cleaning cloths say that the cloths eliminate or mitigate the need for cleaning chemicals. Realistically, crews often can enhance their cleaning efforts in restrooms by applying the appropriate chemicals during the cleaning process.

Powered Cleaning Equipment

Specialized power washers for cleaning restrooms have been available for several years now. Generally, the power washer is cart-mounted for carrying limited cleaning supplies and might come in various sizes. Basically, after the floor has been swept, the unit allows the operator to power-wash the restroom from ceiling to floor and to air dry the room before use.

These units have specialized chemicals, applied through a solution pick-up hose, that afford deep cleaning and drying of surfaces without leaving spots, much like an effective dishwashing agent. More advanced units not only can allow an operator to power spray a room but can also pick up the residue solution after cleaning to minimize the time that a restroom is out of service.

When using these units, operators need use all appropriate safety precautions. For example, crews should not spray chemicals into electrical outlets, and they should make sure that paper goods are adequately protected from solution overspray. When used correctly, these units really do deliver deep cleaning to restrooms.

Manufacturers have provided a new generation of equipment for housekeeping managers to specify to improve the level of restroom cleaning in their facilities. Several can help minimize the use of chemicals.

To complement this cleaning process, Green Seal has developed a "Checklist: Green Seal defines a superior cleaning chemical as "one that lessens its environmental impacts at every stage of its life cycle, including its packaging." Among the items on the checklist are the following:

— Products should be both biodegradable and non-toxic.

— Phosphates concentration should be 5 percent of weight or less, and those without are best.

— Products should work in cold water and be concentrated.

— Avoid products with chlorine bleach or sodium hypochlorite.

— When diluted, concentrations of volatile organic chemicals should not exceed 10 percent of the weight.

— Avoid ingredients that are derived from petroleum.

— Choose surfactants derived from vegetable oil. Avoid those with nonylphenol ethoxylate.

— Use products with a neutral pH.

— Choose products that are packaged in recycled containers.

In addition to this information, the U.S. Environmental Protection Agency (EPA) has developed a Database of Environmental Information for Products and Services. The database provides "useful sources of information on the environmental preferability of products and services.

Housekeeping managers who want to curtail complaints concerning their facilities' restrooms and minimize the impact of cleaning chemicals and processes on the environment have more options than ever today. They can achieve these goals by learning about those options.

Today's environmentally friendly chemicals and equipment are increasingly cost competitive, have increased efficacy, limit damage to the environment and minimize costs to an organization for disposal of chemicals. In more cases than ever, it is a winning combination to clean restrooms with green chemicals and equipment that can solve restroom cleaning complaints and control costs at the same time.

Practices of Infection Control

Housekeeping practices, if performed correctly through educational presentations, will create an area suitable for patient, visitor and healthcare worker to enter and be comfortable within the confines of the environment. The proper maintenance of a health care facility increases the awareness of other employees of the necessity of good sanitary practices. Good housekeeping practices increase moral and public relations. No one wants to work in an area that smells or is dirty.

Sanitation depends upon cleaning thoroughness. There should be procedures in writing to fit each area of the facility such as walls, floors, windows, beds, furniture, draperies, carpets, waste containers, bathrooms, equipment, stairs, elevators, special-care equipment and handling of infectious waste for disposal. Some guideline for infection control are given below:

Patient Rooms

— All horizontal surfaces are cleaned daily or as needed with a registered disinfectant.

— Uncarpeted floors are cleaned daily or as needed with a registered disinfectant.

— Carpeted floors should be vacuumed daily or as needed according to manufacturer's recommendations. Procedures should be spelled out concerning disinfecting carpets that contain blood. The vacuum cleaner should be one that does not add airborne organisms to the environment. Change filters as needed.

— Bathroom is cleaned daily or as needed. Remember that this area of the patient's room may contain high concentrations of body fluids that may neutralize the disinfectant being used.

— Sanitary procedures are performed with common sense in mind.

— Drapes are examined for body fluids or soiling. They do not have to be removed from isolation rooms once the patient has either recovered or been placed in a different locale unless body soils are visible. Drapes have never been implicated in cross contamination of patients.

— Walls are only spot cleaned. There is absolutely no need in washing walls after a patient has been dismissed from a room intended for any type of isolation.

— Normal disinfection procedures are employed in cleaning rooms used for isolation.

— If a patient is in isolation such as airborne, then the appropriate masks should be worn upon entering room.

— Gowns and gloves are used accordingly.

— All patient use items (wheelchairs, etc.) should be disinfected with an EPA registered disinfectant as needed.

— Stainless steel double-bucket system should be used in all areas of the facility. Plastic buckets tend to become soiled and difficult to clean.

— All waste paper baskets should be lined with a plastic bag.

— Housekeeping personnel should report to the executive housekeepers any equipment that is not functioning correctly.

— Make certain that all MSDS forms are up to date.

Other Areas

— Entrances, lobbies, waiting rooms, hallways should be cleaned on a regular schedule or as needed depending on traffic.

— A disinfectant solutions is not really needed in these areas.

— Clean carpets according to manufacturer's recommendations. Make certain that you have discussed with the manufacturer that if blood is spilled on these carpets, what type of chemicals can be used without damaging the fabric. Remember that you must use a tuberculocidal disinfectant on blood spills.

— Examine walls for soilage. Spot clean any wall that contains soil.

Personnel

— Personnel should be free of skin lesions such as herpes, boils, etc.

— All employees in housekeeping should be educated on what requires work restriction due to illness.

— All housekeeping personnel should be ideally vaccinated against tetanus, hepatitis B and influenza.

The chickenpox vaccine is now available for those without prior history of exposure or immunity.

— Rubella and measles vaccine should be part of the employee's responsibility prior to employment.

Regulated Trash

— All housekeeping personnel should be cognizant on what types of waste require regulation. OSHA has defined what requires regulation. However, states, city's and county's may have additional requirements. They should be listed in the procedure manual.

— All housekeeping personnel should have inservice education on Standard Precautions (formerly Universal Precautions) on a yearly basis. Documentation of such education should be made available to any licensing agency.

SUMMATION

— Contamination of the environment is only a risk to the patient if there is a potential mode of transmission.

— Housekeeping is responsible for selecting a disinfectant, writing procedures on how to dilute it and when it should be changed during usage.

— Housekeeping personnel need yearly inservices on infection control practices.

— Cleaning in wrong sequences (soiled to clean) may increase the chance of microbial contamination.

— Use of dry-dusting increases aerosols.

— Use of reusable rather than disposable gloves affords the housekeeper more protection.

— Never store mops in a wet condition. This will increase proliferation of organisms. They should be dried after cleaning.

— Always check with other areas of the hospital/nursing home tomake certain that everyone is doing their job correctly, i.e., surgery, nursery, dietary, etc.

— Make certain that housekeepers understand how to pickup sharps from the floor, i.e., needles.

— Housekeepers must be provided the appropriate barrier protection for their tasks, instructions on where they are located, how to take them off and where to place them after removal.

— All filters in rooms should be checked on a regular schedule. When a filter is removed (changed) from a particular area, the date of newly installed filter should be written clearly on its side with a marking pen. This will enable the housekeeper to determine how often these filters should be changed.

— Change curtains as needed.

— Clean blinds as needed.

— It is not necessary to discard toilet paper or paper towels following patient discharge regardless of the sickness unless they are visibly soiled with body fluids.

— Always make certain that paper towel dispensers are full and that soap dispensers are functional.

— Always check needle disposal boxes to make certain that they are not more than 3/4 full.

— Check to make certain that all screens are functioning correctly.

— Check schedules of waste pickup to make certain that excessive accumulation does not exist.

Every hospital/nursing homes must have in place a written procedure on the type of methods that will be employed to protect the highly susceptible patient from aerosols created during construction projects.

Environment Friendly Cleanliness

The objective of cleaning and sanitizing food contact surfaces is to remove food (nutrients) which bacteria need to grow, and to kill those bacteria which are present. It is important that the clean, sanitized equipment and surfaces drain dry and are stored dry soas to prevent bacteria growth. Necessary equipment must also be clean and stored in a clean, sanitary manner.

Cleaning/sanitizing procedures must be evaluated for adequacy through evaluation and inspection procedures. Adherence to prescribed written procedures (inspection, swab testing, direct observation of personnel) should be continuously monitored, and records maintained evaluate long-term compliance.

The correct order of events for cleaning/ sanitizing of food product contact surfaces is:

— Rinse

— Clean

— Rinse

— Sanitize.

Cleaning is the complete removal of food soil using appropriate detergent chemicals under recommended conditions. It is important that personnel involved have a working understanding of the nature of the different types of food soil and the chemistry of its removal.

Methods

Equipment can be categorized with regard to cleaning method as follows:

— *Mechanical Cleaning*: Often referred to as clean- in-place (CIP) . Require no disassembly or partial disassembly.

— *Clean-out-of-Place (COP)*: Can be partially disassembled and cleaned in specialized COP pressure tanks.
— *Manual Cleaning*: Requires total disassembly for cleaning and inspection.

Sanitization

It is important to differentiate and define certain terminology:

— *Sterilize* refers to the statistical destruction and removal of all living organisms.
— *Disinfect* refers to inanimate objects and the destruction of all vegetative cells (not spores).
— *Sanitize* refers to the reduction of microorganisms to levels considered safe from a public health viewpoint.

Appropriate and approved sanitization procedures are processes and, thus, the duration or time as well as the chemical conditions must be described. The official definition of sanitizing for food product contact surfaces is a process which reduces the contamination level by 99.999% (5 logs) in 30 sec.

The official definition for non-product contact surfaces requires a contamination reduction of 99.9% (3 logs). The standard test organisms used are: Staphylococcus aureus and Escherichia coli. General types of sanitization include:

— *Thermal Sanitization* involves the use of hot water or steam for a specified temperature and contact time.
— *Chemical Sanitization* involves the use of an approved chemical sanitizer at a specified concentration and contact time.

Water Chemistry and Quality

Water comprises approximately 95-99% of cleaning and sanitizing solutions. Water functions to:

— carry the detergent or the sanitizer to the surface

— carry soils or contamination from the surface.

The impurities in water can drastically alter the effectiveness of a detergent or a sanitizer. Water hardness is the most important chemical property with a direct effect on cleaning and sanitizing efficiency. Water pH ranges generally from pH 5 to 8.5. This range is of no serious consequence to most detergents and sanitizers. However, highly alkaline or highly acidic water may require additional buffering agents.

Water can also contain significant numbers of microorganisms. Water used for cleaning and sanitizing must be potable and pathogen-free.

Food Soils

Food soil is generally defined as unwanted matter on food-contact surfaces. Soil is visible or invisible. The primary source of soil is from the food product being handled. However, minerals from water residue and residues from cleaning compounds contribute to films left on surfaces. Microbiological biofilms also contribute to the soil buildup on surfaces.

Since soils vary widely in composition, no one detergent is capable of removing all types. Many complex films contain: combinations of food components, surface oil or dust, insoluble cleaner components, and insoluble hard-water salts. These films vary in their solubility properties depending upon such factors as heat effect, age, dryness, time, etc.

It is essential that personnel involved have an understanding of the nature of the soil to be removed before selecting a detergent or cleaning regime. Therule of thumb is that acid cleaners dissolve alkaline soils (minerals) and alkaline cleaners dissolve acid soils and food wastes. Improper use of detergents can actually "set" soils, making them more difficult to remove (e.g., acid cleaners can precipitate protein). Many films and biofilms require more sophisticated cleaners which are amended with oxidizing agents (such as chlorinated detergents) for removal.

Soils may be classified as:

— soluble in water (sugars, some starches, most salts);

— soluble in acid (limestone and most mineral deposits);

— soluble in alkali (protein, fat emulsions);

— soluble in water, alkali, or acid.

The physical condition of the soil deposits also effects its solubility. Freshly precipitated soil in a cool or cold solution is usually more easily dissolved than an old, dried, or baked-on deposit, or a complex film. Food soils are complex in that they contain mixtures of several components.

Fat

Fat usually is present as an emulsion and can generally be rinsed away with hot water above the melting point. More difficult fat and oil residues can be removed with alkaline detergents which have good emulsifying or saponifying ingredients.

Protein

In the food industry, proteins are by far the most difficult soils to remove. In fact, casein (a major milk protein) is used for its adhesive properties in many glues and paints. Food proteins range from more simple proteins, which are easy to remove, to more complex proteins, which are very difficult to remove. Heat-denatured proteins can be extremely difficult.

Generally, a highly alkaline detergent with peptizing or dissolving properties is required to remove protein soils. Wetting agents can also be used to increase the wettability and suspendability of proteins. Protein films require alkaline cleaners which have hypochlorite in addition to wetting agents.

Carbohydrate

Simple sugars are readily soluble in warm water and are quite easily removed. Starch residues, individually, are also easily removed with mild detergents. Starches associated with proteins or fatscan usually be easily removed by highly alkaline detergents.

Mineral Salt

Mineral salts can be either relatively easy to remove, or be highly troublesome deposits or films. Calcium and magnesium are involved in some of the most difficult mineral films. Under conditions involving heat and alkaline pH, calcium and magnesium can combine with bicarbonates to form highly insoluble complexes. Other difficult deposits contain iron or manganese.

Salt films can also cause corrosion of some surfaces. Difficult salt films require an acid cleaner (especially organic acids which form complexes with these salts) for removal. Sequestering agents such as phosphates or chelating agents are often used in detergents for salt film removal.

Microbiological films

Under certain conditions, microorgranisms (bacteria, yeasts, and molds) can form invisible films (biofilms) on surfaces. Biofilms can be difficult to remove and usually require cleaners as well as sanitizers with strong oxidizing properties.

Lubricating greases and oils

These deposits (insoluble in water, alkali, or acid) can often be melted with hot water or steam, but oftenleave a residue. Surfactants can be used to emulsify the residue to make it suspendable in water and flushable.

Other Insoluble soils

Inert soils such as sand, clay, or fine metal can be removed by surfactant-based detergents. Charred or carbonized material may require organic solvents.

Quantity of Soil

It is important to rinse food-contact surfaces prior to cleaning to remove most of the soluble soil. Heavy deposits require more detergent to remove. Improper cleaning can actually contribute to build-up of soil.

Surface Characteristics

The cleanability of the surface is a primary consideration in evaluating cleaning effectiveness. Included in surface characteristics are:

— *Surface Composition*: Stainless steel is the preferred surface for food equipment and is specified in many industry and regulatory design and construction standards. For example: 3-A Sanitary Standards (equipment standards used for milk and milk products applications) specify 300 series stainless steel or equivalent. Other grades of stainless steel may be appropriate for specific applications (i.e 400 series) such as handling of high fat products, meats, etc. For highly acidic, high salt, or other highly corrosive products, more corrosion resistant materials (i.e. titanium) is often recommended.

Other "soft" metals (aluminum, brass, copper, or mild steel), or nonmetallic surfaces (plastics, or rubber) are also used on food contact surfaces. Surfaces of soft metals and nonmetallic materials are generally less corrosion- resistant and care should be exercised in their cleaning.

Aluminum is readily attacked by acids as well as highly alkaline cleaners which can render the surface non-cleanable. Plastics are subject to stress cracking and clouding from prolonged exposure to corrosive food materials or cleaning agents.

Hard wood (maple or equivalent) or sealed wood surfaces should only be used in limited applications such as cutting boards or cutting tables provided the surface is maintained in good repair. Avoid using porous wood surfaces.

— *Surface Finish*: Equipment design and construction standards also specify finish and smoothness requirements. 3-A standards specify a finish at least as smooth as a No. 4 ground finish for most application. With high-fat products, a less smooth surface is used to allow product release from the surface.

— *Surface Condition*: Misuse or mishandling can result in pitted, cracked, corroded, or roughened surfaces. Such surfaces are more difficult to clean or sanitize, and may no longer be cleanable. Thus, care should be exercised in using corrosive chemicals or corrosive food products.

Environmental Considerations

Detergents can be significant contributors to the waste discharge(effluent). Of primary concern is pH. Many publicly owned treatment works limit effluent pH to the range of 5 to 8.5. So, it is recommended that in applications where highly alkaline cleaners are used, that the effluent be mixed with rinse water (or some other method be used) to reduce the pH. Recycling of caustic soda cleaners is also becoming a common practice in larger operations. Other concerns are phosphates, which are not tolerated in some regions of the U.S., and the overall soil load in the waste stream which contributes to the chemical oxygen demand (COD) and biological oxygen demand (BOD).

Chemistry of Detergents

Detergents and cleaning compounds are usually composed of mixtures of ingredients that interact with soils in several ways:

— Physically active ingredients alter physical characteristics such as solubility or colloidal stability.

— Chemically active ingredients modify soil components to make them more soluble and, thus, easier to remove.

In some detergents, specific enzymes are added to catalytically react with, and degrade, specific food soil components.

Physically active ingredients

The primary physically active ingredients are the surface active compounds termed surfactants. These organic molecules have general structural characteristicwhere a portion of the structure is hydrophilic (water- loving) and a portion is hydrophobic (not reactive with water). Such molecules function in detergents by promoting the physical cleaning actions through: emulsification, penetration, spreading, foaming, and wetting. The classes of surfactants are:

— *Ionic surfactants* which are negatively charged in water solution are termed anionic surfactants. Conversely, positively charged ionic surfactants are termed cationic surfactants. If the charge of the water soluble portion is depended upon the pH of the solution it is termed an amphoteric surfactant. These surfactants behave as cationic surfactants under acid conditions, and as anionic surfactants under alkaline conditions. Ionic surfactants are generally characterized by their high foaming ability.

— *Nonionic surfactants* , which do not dissociate when dissolved in water, have the broadest range of properties depending upon the ratio of hydrophilic/hydrophobic balance. This balance is also affected by temperature. For example, the foaming properties of nonionic detergents is affected by temperature of solution. As temperature increases, the hydrophobic character and solubility decreases. At the cloud point (minimum solubility), these surfactants generally act as defoamers, while below the cloud point they are varied in their foaming properties.

It is a common practice to blend surfactant ingredients to optimize their properties. However, because of precipitation problems, cationic and anionic surfactants cannot be blended

Chemically active ingredients

Alkaline Builders: *Highly Alkaline Detergents (or heavy-duty detergents)* use caustic soda (sodium hydroxide) or caustic potash (potassium hydroxide). An important property of these highly alkaline detergents is that they saponify fats: forming soap. These cleaners are used in many CIP systems or bottle-washing applications.

Moderately Alkaline Detergents include sodium, potassium, or ammonium salts of phosphates, silicates, or carbonates. Tri-sodium phosphate (TSP) is one of the oldest and most effective. Silicates are most oftenused as a corrosion inhibitor. Because of interaction with calcium and magnesium and film formation, carbonate-based detergents are of only limited use in food processing cleaning regimes.

Acid Builders: *Acid Detergents* include organic and inorganic acids. The most common inorganic acids used include: phosphoric, nitric, sulfamic, sodium acid sulfate, and hydrochloric. Organic acids, such as hydroxyacetic, citric, and gluconic, are also in use. Acid detergents are often used in a two-step sequential cleaning regime with alkaline detergents. Acid detergents are also used for the prevention or removal of stone films (mineral stone, beer stone, or milk stone).

Water Conditioners: Water conditioners are used to prevent the build-up of various mineral deposits (water hardness, etc.). These chemicals are usually sequestering agents or chelating agents. Sequestering agents form soluble complexes with calcium and magnesium. Examples are sodium tripolyphosphate, tetra-potassium pyrophosphate, organo-phosphates, and polyelectrolytes. Chelating agents include sodium gluconate and ethylene diamine tetracetic acid (EDTA).

Oxidizing agents: Oxidizing agents used in detergent application are hypochlorite (also a sanitizer) and--to a lesser extent -- perborate. Chlorinated detergents are most often used to clean protein residues.

Enzyme Ingredients

Enzyme-based detergents, which are amended with enzymes such as amylases and other carbohydrate-degrading enzymes, proteases, and lipases, are finding acceptance in specialized food industry applications.

The primary advantages of enzyme detergents are that they are more environmentally friendly and often require less energy input (less hot water in cleaning). Uses of most enzyme cleaners are usually limited to unheated surfaces (e.g., cold-milk surfaces). However, new generation enzyme cleaners (currently under evaluation) are expected to have broader application.

Fillers

Fillers add bulk or mass, or dilute dangerous detergent formulations which are difficult to handle. Strong alkalis are often diluted with fillers for ease and safety of handling. Water is used in liquid formulations as a filler. Sodium chloride or sodium sulfate are often fillers in powdered detergent formuations.

Miscellaneous Ingredients

Additional ingredients added to detergents may include: corrosion inhibitors, glycol ethers, and butylcellosolve (improve oil, grease, and carbon removal).

Sanitizing

Thermal Sanitizing

As with any heat treatment, the effectiveness of thermal sanitizing is dependant upon a number of factors including: initial contamination load, humidity, pH, temperature, and time.

Steam

The use of steam as a sanitizing process has limited application. It is generally expensive compared to alternatives, and it is difficult to regulate and monitor contact temperature and time. Further, the byproducts of steam condensation can complicate cleaning operations.

Hot Water Sanitizing

Hot-water sanitizing--through immersion (small parts, knives, etc.), spray (dishwashers), or circulating systems--is commonly used. The time required is determined by the temperature of the water. Typical regulatory requirements (Food Code 1995) for use of hot water in dishwashing and utensil sanitizing applications specify: immersion for at least 30 sec. at 77°C (170°F) for manual operations; a final rinse temperature of 74°C (165°F) in single tank, single temperature machines and 82°C (180°F) for other machines.

Many state regulations require a utensil surface temperature of 71°C (160°F) as measured by an irreversibly registering temperature indicator in warewashing machines. Recommendations andrequirements for hot-water sanitizing in food processing may vary. The Grade A Pasteurized Milk Ordinance specifies a minimum of 77°C (170°F) for 5 min. Other recommendations for processing operations are: 85°C (185°F) for 15 min., or 80°C (176°F) for 20 min.

The primary advantages of hot-water sanitization are: relatively inexpensive, easy to apply and readily available, generally effective over a broad range of microorganisms, relatively non-corrosive, and penetratesinto cracks and crevices. Hot-water sanitization is a slow process which requires come-up and cool-down time; can have high energy costs; and has certain safety concerns for employees. The process also has the disadvantages of forming or contributing to film formations, and shortening the life of certain equipment or parts thereof (gaskets, etc.).

Chemical Sanitizing

The ideal chemical sanitizer should:

— be approved for food contact surface application

— have a wide range or scope of activity.

— destroy microorganisms rapidly.

— be stable under all types of conditions.

— be tolerant of a broad range of environmental conditions.

— be readily solubilized and possess some detergency.

— be low in toxicity and corrosivity.

— be inexpensive.

No available sanitizer meets all of the above criteria. Therefore, it is important to evaluate the properties, advantages, and disadvantages of available sanitizer for each specific application.

Regulatory considerations

The regulatory concerns involved with chemical sanitizers are: antimicrobial activity or efficacy, safety of residues on food contact surfaces, and environmental safety. It is important to follow regulations that apply for each chemical usage situation. The registration of chemical sanitizers and antimicrobial agents for use on food and food product contact surfaces, and on nonproduct contact surfaces, is through the U.S. Environmental Protection Agency (EPA). (Prior to approval and registration, the EPAreviews efficacy and safety data, and product labeling information.

The U.S. Food and Drug Administration (FDA) is primarily involved in evaluating residues form sanitizer use which may enter the food supply. Thus, any antimicrobial agent and its maximum usage level for direct use on food or on food product contact surfaces must be approved by the FDA. Approved no-rinse food contact sanitizes and nonproduct contact sanitzers, their formulations and usage levels are listed in the Code of Federal Regulations.

The U.S. Department of Agriculture (USDA) also maintains lists of antimicrobial compounds (i.e., USDA List of Proprietary Substances and Non Food Product Contact Compounds) which are primarily used in the regulation of meats, poultry, and related products by USDA's Food Safety and Inspection Service (FSIS.).

Sanitizer Effectiveness

Physical factors

Surface Characteristics: Prior to the sanitization process, all surfaces must be clean and thoroughly rinsed to remove any detergent residue. An unclean surface cannot be sanitized. Since the effectiveness of sanitization requires direct contact with the microorganisms, the surface should be free of cracks, pits, or crevices which can harbor microorganisms. Surfaces which contain biofilms cannot be effectively sanitized.

Exposure Time: Generally, the longer time a sanitizer chemical is in contact with the equipment surface, the more effective the sanitization effect; intimate contact is as important as prolonged contact..

Temperature: Temperature is also positively related to microbial kill by a chemical sanitizer. Avoid high temperatures (above 55°C [131°F]) because of the corrosive nature of most chemical sanitizers.

Concentration: Generally, the activity of a sanitizer increases with increased concentration. However, a leveling off occurs at high concentrations. A common misconception regarding chemicals is that "if a little is good, more is better". Using sanitizer concentrations above recommendations does not sanitizer better and, in fact, can be corrosive to equipment and in the long run lead to less cleanability. Follow manufacturer's label instructions.

Soil: The presence of organic matter dramatically reduces the activity of sanitizers and may, in fact, totally inactivate them. The adage is "you cannot sanitize an unclean surface".

Chemical factors

pH: Sanitizers are dramatically affected by the pH of the solution. Many chlorine sanitizers, for example, are almost ineffective at pH values above 7.5.

Water properties: Certain sanitizers are markedly affected by impurities in the water.

Inactivators: Organic and/or inorganic inactivators may react chemically with sanitizers giving rise to non-germicidal products. Some of these inactivators are present in detergent residue. Thus, it is important that surfaces be rinsed prior to sanitization.

Biological factors

The microbiological load can affect sanitizer activity. Also, the type of microorganism present is important. Spores are more resistant than vegetative cells. Certain sanitizers are more active against gram positive than gram negative microorganisms, and vice versa. Sanitizers also vary in their effectiveness against yeasts, molds, fungi, and viruses.

Types of Chemical Sanitizers

The chemicals described here are those approved by FDA for use as no-rinse, food-contact surface sanitizers. In food-handling operations, these are used as rinses, sprayed onto surfaces, or circulated through equipment in CIP operations. In certain applications the chemicals are foamed on a surface or fogged into the air to reduce airborne contamination.

Chlorine-based sanitizers

Chlorine Compounds: Chlorine, in its various forms, is the most commonly used sanitizer in food processing and handling applications. Commonly used chlorine compounds include: liquid chlorine, hypochlorites, inorganic chloramines, and organic chloramines. Chlorine-based sanitizers form hypochlorous acid (HOCl, the most active form) in solution. Available chlorine (the amount of HOCl present) is a function of pH. At pH 5, nearly all is in the form of HOCl. At pH 7.0, approximately 75% is HOCl.

The maximumallowable level for no-rinse applications is 200ppm available chlorine, but recommended usage levels vary. For hypochlorites, an exposure time of 1 min at a minimum concentration of 50ppm and a temperature of 24°C (75°F) is recommended. For each 10°C (18°F) drop in temperature, a doubling of exposure time is recommended. For chloramines, 200ppm for 1 min is recommended.

Chlorine compounds are broad spectrum germicides which act on microbial membranes, inhibit cellular enzymes involved in glucose metabolism, have a lethal effect on DNA, and oxidize cellular protein. Chlorine has activity at low temperature, is relatively cheap, and leaves minimal residue or film on surfaces. The activity of chlorine is dramatically affected by such factors as pH, temperature, and organic load. However, chlorine is less affected by water hardness when compared to other sanitizers.

The major disadvantage to chlorine compound is corrosiveness to many metal surfaces. Health and safety concerns can occur due to skin irritation and mucous membrane damage in confined areas. At low pH (below 4.0), deadly Cl_2 (mustard gas) can form. In recent years, concerns have also been raised about the use of chlorine as a drinking water disinfectant and as an antimicrobial with direct food contact (meat, poultry and shellfish).

This concern is based upon the involvement of chlorine in the formation of potentially carcinogenic trihalomethanes (THMs) under appropriate conditions. While chlorine's benefits as a sanitizer far outweigh these risks, it is under scrutiny.

Chlorine dioxide: Chlorine dioxide (ClO_2) is currently being considered as a replacement for chlorine, since it appears to be more environmentally friendly. Stabilized ClO_2 has FDA approval for most applications in sanitizing equipment or for use as a foam for environmental and non-food contact surfaces. Approval has also been granted for use in flume waters in fruits and vegetable operations and in poultry process waters.

ClO_2 has 2.5 times the oxidizing power of chlorine and, thus, less chemical is required. Typical use concentrations range from 1to 10ppm. ClO_2's primary disadvantages are worker safety and toxicity. Its highly concentrated gases can be explosive and exposure risks to workers is higher thanthat for chlorine. Its rapid decomposition in the presence of light, or at temperatures greater than 50°C (122°F) makes on-site generation a recommended practice.

Iodine

Use of iodine as an antimicrobial agents dates back to the 1800s. This sanitizer exists in many forms and usually exists with a surfactant as a carrier. These mixtures are termed iodophors. The most active agent is the dissociated free iodine. This form is most prevalent at low pH. The amount of dissociation from the surfactant is dependent upon the type of surfactant. Iodine solubility is very limited in water. Generally recommended usage for iodophors is 12.5 to 25ppm for 1 min.

It is generally thought that the bactericidal activity of iodine is through direct halogenation of proteins. More recent theories have centered upon cell wall damage and destruction of microbial enzyme activity. Iodophors, like chlorine compounds, have a very broad spectrum: being active against bacteria, viruses, yeasts, molds, fungi, and protozoans. Iodine is highly temperature-dependent and vaporizes at 120°F. Thus, it is limited to lower temperature applications.

The degree to which iodophors are affected by environmental factors is highly dependant upon properties of the surfactant used in the formulation. Iodophors are generally less affected by organic matter and water hardness than chlorine. However, loss of activity is pronounced at high pH. Iodine has a long history of use in wound treatment. However, ingestion of iodine gas does pose a toxicity risk in closed environments. The primary disadvantage is that iodine can cause staining on some surfaces (especially plastics).

7

Floor Maintenance

Maintaining floors involves a long program consisting of multiple steps. First step starts with the cutting of extra-unwanted things that are glued to the floor with the help of a sharp edged knife. While cleaning, don't forget to clean those areas especially which are left out on a daily basis. One out of ten days should be kept for extra cleaning with a broom reaching out those areas, which remain untouched. Pick up a nice clean duster and get ready for the dusting work. Wipe off all the dust.

Maintenance for Hardwood Floors

How to care for hardwood floor surface that requires special maintenance. These steps suggest ways to make your hardwood floors last longer. Hardwood floors require special care to keep them in beautiful conditions. Many people choose hard floors because they believe it is easier to care for them than carpets. This can be true, but it depends on the materials of which the floor is made.

A hardwood floor can be made from many different kinds of wood. Oak is the wood of choice because it is hard and attractively grained. Maple, walnut, and teak are also popular, but more expensive than oak. Softer woods such as pine are sometimes used in areas that are not as frequently seen. Soft woods are more easily dented and scratched.

Wood is porous and absorbent, which makes them especially susceptible to water damage. Anyone cleaning the floor must avoid alkaline substances such as sudsy cleaners or ammonia as they can cause dark spots. If the dark spots appear, they can be removed with vinegar applications. There are many ways that wood can be laid on a floor. Parquet floors are made of wood tiles, often of different colors, that are laid in a geometric pattern or mosaic. They are usually oak or maple. Wood block floors are shaped like butcher block surfaces and also come in tiles. Plank floors are long strips of wood that are fitted together to make a smooth appearance.

Regular cleaning and finishing of hardwood floors will help them retain their appearance and durability. Before starting to clean, you should gather all the equipment you will need. This may include a broom or dust mop, a dustpan, floor wax, a cloth, and a buffer machine with pads. Clear the floor of movable furniture or other items. Sweep or dust-mop the area. By removing all loose dirt before waxing, you are preventing dirty wax buildup. Do not use water to clean the floors. Water on wood floors can damage the wood and cause wax to turn milky white. If you have a white spot caused by water, you can remove it by rubbing a small amount of mineral spirits into the spot with a fine steel wool.

You should also be careful not to over-treat mops because the chemical on the mop head will transfer to the floor. This can create a haze or dulling effect and may even destroy the finish. Mop heads come in a variety of natural or synthetic fibers. If you think there is too much chemical on the mop head, soak it in water for 30 minutes before using it. It also helps to soak new mop heads to get rid of any sizing chemicals they have.

Most hardwood floor care experts recommend sweeping or dust-mopping on a daily basis. Dirt particles on a floor can scratch the surface when you or others walk on it. Waxing also strengthens wood surfaces and other porous floor materials. The most efficient way to wax a floor is through buffing or burnishing.

Buffing involves spraying the floor with a polishing solution and buffing the floor with a rotary floor machine. Check the electrical cords on the buffer machine and make sure the cords are untangled and free of damage. Attach a buffer pad to the buffer machine and work small amounts of wax into the buffer machine pad with your fingers or a cloth. Buff the floor until it shines.

Burnishing is a slightly newer method of cleaning floors. It is similar to buffing, except that it is a dry method. It also uses a rotary floor machine, but it uses a faster rotation on the machine head.

If there are stains on the floor, you will need to do the following:

— Identify the stain and determine how to treat it.
— Remove solid particles with a hand-held scraper, being careful not to scratch or gouge the floor.
— Use a wet vacuum on large wet stains.
— Spot-test the stain remover and apply it according to the manufacturer's direction.

Clean and Wax Tile Floors

Clean and wax tile floors with thses easy tips for different surface types and proper care. There are many types of tile floors, with the most common ones being vinyl, linoleum, and ceramic. While the latter does not require waxing, the other two types of floors do. Floor-care experts even recommend waxing the "no-wax" floors as it can protect the surface from abrasion.

Vinyl floors are made of pure vinyl or a blend of vinyl and another material. The pure vinyl floors usually cost twice as much as vinyl blend floors. Vinyl resists most stains and substances. Vinyls with a cushioned backing have extra resiliency and absorb noise. Overall, it is an easy surface to care for.

Linoleum can be made from a variety of materials, typically linseed oil, ground cork or wood, resins, and mineral fillers. It is often bonded to a burlap or felt backing for extra resilience or strength. It is inexpensive, easy to install, and easy to maintain. However, strong detergents will damage it.

Ceramic tile is made from clay, marble, slate, glass, or flint. It is very durable and easy to maintain.

Before starting to clean, gather everything you will need. To clean and wax tile floors you may need any or all of the following: a broom or dust-mop, a buffer machine with brushes or pads, detergent, stripping chemical, white vinegar, a floor sealer, floor wax, a putty knife, cleaning cloths, a wrung-out mop or wet vacuum, a mop bucket, a mop for wet mopping, a dustpan, latex gloves, protective goggles, a bucket, a spray bottle and a small brush.

Begin by sweeping or dust mopping the area. You'll need to clear the floor of all furniture or other objects. Remove all loose dust and dirt by using a broom or a clean, dry dust mop and dustpan.

Methods of Stains Removal from the Floor

Wet-mop tile floors on a weekly or as-needed basis. Select the appropriate cleaner for the type of floor that you have. There are two methods you can use for mopping a floor.

Method 1

Mix the cleaner with water in the mop bucket and apply

it to the floor. Dump the dirty water and refill the mop bucket with clean rinse water. Mop the floor with rinse water, changing the water as needed. Wring the mop and soak up excess water so the floor is just damp.

Method 2

Mix the appropriate cleaner and water in a spray bottle. Fill the mop bucket with clean rinse water. Spray the floor with the cleaner. Dip the mop in the rinse bucket, wring the mop and mop up the cleaning solution.

Whichever method you use, start in the back of the room away from the door or entrance hallway. Mop from left to right in three-foot sections, working toward the door. Each three-foot section should overlap the previous one. Working from the back of the room to the front and overlapping mopped sections will prevent you from walking on the cleaned area and will make sure that the entire floor area is clean.

Let the floor air dry. Empty the mop bucket, rinse it with clean water, and hang it to dry. Rinse the mop in clean water and hang it to dry.

Floors will occasionally need to be stripped and refinished. Stripping removes all of the old floor finish and the dirt that has been ground into the finish. Waxing the floor puts on a sealer or finish that protects the floor from wear and staining. It also should make the floor more slip resistant.

Floor care experts suggest that the following signs mean it is time to refinish a floor:

1. There are worn traffic areas showing and the bare floor is becoming exposed through worn-away finish or sealer.
2. The finish has an obvious flaking or chipping.

3. The floor is no longer shiny and has dark shadowy areas.
4. Spills have stained the floor.
5. There is built-up wax on the floor. Built-up wax may look yellow or have gray or black patches.

The first step in refinishing a floor is to strip the floor. After the floor has been stripped, it should be completely clean and ready to receive a new wax coat.

Wear heavy latex utility gloves and protective goggles when stripping built-up wax or sealer from tile floors. Mix water and an ammonia-based floor stripper. Apply a heavy coat of the ammonia solution with a mop. Let this stand for 10 minutes or until a haze appears.

Hand-scrub the edges with a brush. Scrape the wax loose from corners with a small putty knife. Pick up residue in corners and along edges with a hand cloth if needed. Scrub the wax loose use a buffer machine with a brush or nylon pads.

Use a warm, clean rinse water and a wet vacuum or a wrung-out mop to pick up wax and dirt. Change the rinse water as needed. Add one cup of white vinegar to 2.5 gallons of rinse water. Use this solution as a final rinse to get rid of any film from the wax and stripping solution. Be sure to reach corners and edges. Air dry the floor.

Using a mop, apply one coat of sealer and three coats of wax. In high-traffic areas, you may need two coats of sealer and three coats of wax. There are two main types of finishes: wax-based and polymer finish. Wax-based polishes require at least two coats of wax. Polymer finishes typically contain a dissolved metal, usually zinc, that strengthens the floor finish. It is a strong finish that is easily touched up to keep the floor glossy. Polymer finishes are also easier to strip.

Apply liquid wax evenly to the clean, dry tile floor. Make even strokes with a little overlap. Wait 30 minutes or longer before going back over missed areas. Apply the next coat at a right angle to the first coat to catch any hairlines missed. If you are just touching up a wax finish, mix half liquid wax and half water in a spray bottle. Spray lightly on the floor just ahead of the buffer machine. Buff until a glossy finish appears.

Rinse all of your mops well and hang them to dry. Clean other supplies and equipment and hang them to dry as necessary. While stripping and refinishing is time-consuming, it can prolong the life of your floor and keep a high quality appearance.

Cleaning Stains from Tile Floor

Cleaning stains from tile floors vary with the type of stain. Follow these tips from professional housekeepers to remove stains and protect your floors.

Stains can challenge even the most creative housekeeper. Fortunately, professional housekeepers have come up with a number of ways to combat stains and keep tile floors looking clean and attractive. Whenever you have to work with strong chemicals or are cleaning up body fluid stains or blood, you should wear heavy latex utility gloves and protective goggles.

Before doing any stain removal process, you should test it. Do this by applying it to a small area of the floor that is out of sight or covered by furniture. If the remover damages the floor, do not continue. It may be necessary to contact the tile manufacturer for instructions.

Blood Stains

Cover the area with paper towels. Pour a fresh solution of phenolic liquid detergent or disinfectant and water on the paper towels. Let the solution stand for 15 minutes. Throw away the paper towels in a sealable plastic container. Wipe the area with dry paper towels. If you do not know whose blood it is or there is a chance that the blood is infected with bloodborne pathogens, you need to take extra precautions.

Bloodborne pathogens are viruses, bacteria, and other microorganisms that are carried in a person's bloodstream and other body fluids. They can cause the Hepatitis B Virus (HBV), the Human Immunodeficiency Virus (HIV), and other infections. Examine the gloves for tears, cracks, and holes before and after use. Do not use damaged gloves. Remove gloves properly and wash your hands. Dispose of the gloves.

Burns

If the burn has destroyed the tile, you will probably have to replace it.

Candy, Chewing Gum, or Candle Wax

Scrape up gum or candy with a putty knife. Apply an all-purpose detergent solution. To remove gum from hard or 100% vinyl resilient tile, use denatured alcohol or a powdered detergent. Rinse the spot with a wet cloth or sponge.

If the gum does not scrape off, try first freezing it to brittleness using ice cubes and then scraping it off with a plastic spatula. There are also commercially available gum removers that can be used on some stains.

Fresh Fruit Stains

Dip a clean cloth into a solution of detergent and warm water. Rub gently. If the floor is a resilient surface (such as vinyl, cork, or wood), mix one tablespoon of oxalic acid and one pint of water, dip the cloth in it and rub again.

Heel Marks

Try using a pencil eraser to remove heel marks. If that doesn't work, rub heel marks with an all-purpose detergent and steel wool. Some experts suggest using a commercial concentrated household cleaner that has a petroleum solvent or using a solvent-based cleaner.

Ink Stains

Clean with a strong all-purpose detergent solution and steel wool. If the stain persists, dampen a cloth with ammonia and place it over the stain for several minutes. Rinse well.

Use denatured alcohol to remove some inks if the stain is on a hard surface or 100% vinyl resilient tile. There are commercially available ink stain removers, but most cannot be used on hard-surfaced floors.

Nail Polish

Blot as much of the polish as possible using a dry cloth of sponge. Clean with all-purpose detergent solution. Apply nail polish remover. Do not use nail polish remover on rubber or asphalt tile. Some experts suggest using baby oil instead of nail polish remover.

Urine Stains

Be sure to wear protective equipment such as goggles and gloves and follow the same procedures as for bloodborne pathogens.

If the stain is fresh, use absorbent paper towels to blot it until you can't soak up any more urine. Use #0 steel wool if necessary and a strong bleach solution. Put the paper towels, steel wool, and gloves in a sealable plastic container before disposing of it. Wash your hands thoroughly as soon as you remove your gloves.

For older stains, dilute liquid bleach in hot water (preferably at a 1:10 mix). Dip a clean cloth into the water and rub the spot. Rinse well with clean water.

No matter what the stain, you may have to strip and wax the floor or touch up the wax finish after removing a stain.

Floor buffing machine

Buffer machines provide that extra shine to hard floors and painted surfaces. Buffer machines serve many purposes. They are used to clean, strip, and wax floors. Smaller buffer machines are used to paint and polish nearly any surface.

Buffer machines can provide that extra shine to hard floors. They can be tricky to use, but once mastered can help you keep your floors in top condition.

Before getting started, check the electrical cords on the buffer machine. They should be untangled and free of damage.

Make sure the machine is unplugged. Tilt it backward until the operating handle rests on the floor. Make sure the scrub brush or pad is clean, or you could end up damaging the floor. Twist the brush or pad on the suds counterclockwise.

Plug in the buffer machine. Buff the floor with the buffer machine, working from the far side of the room to the entrance. Work backward slowly in a fanning motion from left to right. Be sure you have a good grip on the buffer machine as it is easy to lose control of the higher-powered machines. Operate the buffer with one hand, and use your other hand to move the electrical cord out of your path.

Check the pad or brush at set intervals, and change dirty pads or brushes. If a film is left on the floor, you'll need to mop the floor and then buff again using a clean brush or pad on the machine. When you are done buffing, remove the buffer pad or brush from the machine, clean all buffer pads or brushes and hang them to dry. Never leave pads or brushes on the buffer machine.

Professional painters often use buffing machines to polish and buff paint. It is quicker than hand polishing and reduces the expense involved in painting. There are two main kinds of machines that painters use: buffers and orbital polishers. A buffer is a type of body grinder with a polishing pad instead of a grinding disc. Orbital polishers are less powerful, less likely to have variable speed and have a special head that forces the bonnet to run in a variable pattern.

Caution must be used with buffers as their high speed raises the risk that a molding will be popped off, a hole burnt in the paint, or other problems caused.

There are two types of pads: cutting and polishing. Cutting pads are much faster, but they can leave swirl marks on dark finishes. They are usually made of wool, either synthetic or natural. Many experts recommend lamb's wool. Polishing pads are used for finishing. They are made of foam rubber and can be used on almost any surface, including clearcoat finishes.

Whenever using a buffer, you should wear safety goggles. Buff a single section at a time, starting with the least abrasive polish that will be effective. Because most buffers rotate clockwise, you should left the left side of the buffer slightly and move the buffer in smooth left to right strokes. This will help prevent buffer burns and keep the pad always rotating off the edge.

Start slowly and spread the polish evenly across the surface you are buffing. Once the polish has spread, increase the speed slightly. Keep the buffer moving as you work the polish in. Check the pad at set intervals and change it when it becomes caked with polish. Alternatively, you can use a dull screwdriver to clean most pads. Foam pads should be cleaned only with water.

VACUUMING

There is a true art to vacuuming, spend your time on other things yet keep your hotel vacuumed, you can. It is easy. There are many types of vacuum cleaners on the market today but in any case here are a few hints on using that vaccum and its attachments. First of all get one with a powerful enough motor to last and endure all those cleaning tasks for years to come. You can just price and get information before buying your new vacuum.

This is one of the most useful pieces of equipment you will own in your hotel as it can help with so many cleaning tasks. Each vacuum should come with cleaning attachments and these each have various uses. The wand is used when you require extra lenth for cleaning bare floors or hard to reach places. The dusting brush is for furniture, tables tops, books, bookcases, light fixtures, just about anything in your hotel that will get dusty. There should be a floor brush for hard-surfaced polished or waxed floor and for carpet. You might also have a shag rake included for those shag rugs. There will be an upholstery nozzle for the upholestered furniture, sofas, chairs, draperies, and so many other items in the hotel. A crevice toole for upholestered furniture, edges of wall to wall carpeting, those dresser drawers and lots more may be included. The vacuum will also come with a disposable bag, which needs to be changed when full as the vacuum will work less efficiently.

Set the control on the vaccum according to the surface you are cleaning and the degree of suction you might need for that task. On some vacuums, that adjustment might be automatic.

Before you vacuum, check the area to be sure there are not any objects that might get in the vacuum and cause possible harm.

Push the vacuum slowly in straight strokes. This keeps you from going over each section several times to remove deeply embedded soil. As you work, be sure to keep the cord from getting tangled.

Try out the individual nozzles and attachments to see which one might do the very best cleaning job on the task you have selected. Be sure to always check the vacuum bag before beginning. With these few helpful hints your hotel should be very clean and when guests arrive you will be more than proud of your accomplishments.

Types of Vacuums

There are many types of vacuums that people use to clean. Some vacuums are used just for everyday cleaning and other vacuums are used for professional cleaning. The two main types of vacuums are uprights and canisters. Both vacuums have their own benefits and disadvantages.

Upright vacuums

These types of vacuums are good in the fact that they are usually very easy to maneuver around and can be controlled with one hand. They have very powerful motors and are much more durable than other types of vacuums, including the canister. Most professional cleaners prefer to use this type of vacuum as opposed to all other vacuums.

An upright vacuum, however, is not very handy for cleaning up and down stairs, in corners, on upholstery, floors or cleaning far underneath furniture and other things. But for surface carpet cleaning, an upright is the most powerful cleaner around.

Canister vacuums

These types of vacuums are excellent for cleaning up and down stairs, on upholstery, in corners, and everywhere else where the upright vacuum cannot clean well. This vacuum is also the best choice for cleaning floors without carpets. The reason for this is because when you are using an upright to clean a hard surface floor, unless you can stop the brush from spinning as you clean, most of the dust will be scooped up by the brush and shot out the sides or out of the back of the upright vacuum. So if effect, you are not actually cleaning the floor, you are moving the dirt and dust around. The canister vacuum has an attachment for the floor. There is no brush that spins therefore the dirt and dust goes right into the vacuum and the floor gets cleaned.

The canister vacuum usually comes with an assortment of attachment tools for different cleaning jobs. It is easier to use the attachments with a canister vacuum rather than an upright vacuum. Although some upright vacuums do come with attachment tools, when you use the attachments on an upright vacuum, the vacuum tends to fall down from the weight and from pulling on it.

A canister vacuum, unlike the upright, is not the easiest vacuum to maneuver around. Besides the vacuum head to push, you also need to pull the unit behind you and around corners as you vacuum. This tends to cause problems when you want to vacuum around furniture or as you vacuum into different rooms in the hotel.

The attachments that most vacuums come with are used for different jobs. Some vacuums come with so many attachments that it is often difficult to distinguish which attachments are used in which jobs. Most of the attachments that come with upright and canister vacuums have the same general description. There are a few variations but they mostly look the same.

Cleaning your floor tile is no fun unless you know the easy secret of using your kids and big towels. If you have a lot of floor tile, chances are you dread cleaning it. There are many reasons for this. The back and forth motion of the mops on the market today, make for sore arms and backs. If you are the type that loves a really clean floor, your hands and knees have probably been your last resort to get it that way.

Other problems with old methods of cleaning floor tile is that only small surfaces can be cleaned at a time. Marks are left as the surface dries. Another reason for concern is that tile can be very slippery, especially the shiny version. If you have children, cleaning your tile is a real concern because if they happen to walk on it before it dries, it is very easy to slip and fall. Many very serious accidents have been attributed to wet tile.

All you need for cleaning solution is warm water. If your tile is really dirty, you might put a drop or two of dish soap to a gallon of warm water. Use very little if you use any at all. Warm water works the best for most jobs. Make sure the water temperature isn't too hot if you have children helping you

Wet and ring out your towels. This is the hardest part, but it can even be fun if you do it in the bathtub. Have a child stand in each end of a dry tub. Have each child take an end of the wet towel. Have one start to twist the towel one way, the other start to twist the towel the other way.

Each child needs a towel to start the fun of cleaning the tile. Spread the damp towel out on the floor to be cleaned. Have a child step on the towel with feet about a foot apart. The idea then is to shuffle the feet, moving the towel with you as you go. It is fun to have races or see who can shuffle over the largest space in the shortest amount of time. The weight of the body with the shuffling motion of the feet will clean tile very effectively.

After you have gone over the entire floor, repeat the process using dry towels. The floor is dried very quickly. There are no slips, no marks left, and the floor dries to a clean, dry finish in no time. The rags are thrown into the washing machine easily. It's great fun. Children love competitive games. Make it a game. It's amazing how much they will get done.

Cleaning no wax floors

No wax floors are fairly simple to maintain, but they do require some special care to keep them looking new longer. However, this is not a difficult chore. By using a doormat at each entrance of your hotel you will help keep out the dirt and debris that can be tracked in on your shoes. For the best results, place a mat both inside and outside of the doors.

Sweeping and vacuuming regularly is a must. Sweeping the floors every day will get rid of the daily dust that accumulates and will get rid of the dirt and other debris that can wreak havoc on the protective top layer of your no-wax floor. And you should vacuum the floor at least once a week.

Wipe spills off of your floors as soon as possible, using warm water. Dry with a clean cotton or terrycloth towel. If the floor is stained with a stubborn food, beverage or rust stain, cover the stain with a white cotton or terrycloth washcloth saturated with a mild bleach solution. (One capful of bleach to one gallon of water.) Cover and leave on the stain no longer than one hour, then rinse the area thoroughly with water before proceeding to the next step.

For stubborn oil-based stains, ink stains and scuff marks, use a white cotton or terrycloth washcloth saturated with isopropyl alcohol to wipe up the stain, then you'll want to rinse the area thoroughly with water before proceeding to the next step.

To remove paint or nail polish from your floor, you should use alcohol to wipe up the stain. You should then damp mop the floor with a mild solution of ammonia and water. Mix one to three capfuls of ammonia to one gallon of warm water. You may also use a mild solution of vinegar and water. Never use a harsh or abrasive cleaner as this will scratch the surface of the floor. Overdoing the ammonia or vinegar mixture is not a good idea either as it will leave your floors looking dull. Do not use a regular floor wax. Rinsing the floor with a warm water rinse, while not required, will help your floor maintain it's shine. You, then, should dry the floor with a clean white cotton or terrycloth towel. Drying the floor may seem like an unnecessary step, but don't skip it. It will help you maintain an even floor shine.

Every two years, you will need to use a special floor finish to maintain the shine. Check with the flooring manufacturer for special supplies or you may use a floor polish that does not require buffing. Buffing the floor will cause it to lose its shine. Apply two to three coats of floor wax, allowing the floor to dry completely before applying the next coat.

Every four years, you should strip the floor of its old wax to maintain the shine. Check with the manufacturer of the flooring for supplies. With regular care of your no-wax floors, the shine will last for years to come.

Cleaning Ceramic Tiles

Explains how to remove dirt, mold, mildew and water deposits from ceramic tile surfaces using simple cleaning solutions and processes. Ceramic tiles are popular as design features within many areas of today's modern hotels. They vary in size, style, color and cost, and are popularly used because of their beauty as well as their ease to clean. Whether used as flooring or on walls, ceramic tiles can be maintained easily if you follow some standard procedures for their upkeep.

Ceramic tiles are made from clay that contain silicates. To produce a tile, this clay mixture is formed and baked at high temperatures. Ceramic tiles can be purchased in two forms: unglazed or glazed. Unglazed tiles typically require more cleaning maintenance because they are not coated with an outer shell. All tiles, however, can, and should be, routinely cleaned using a plain water solution. By wiping down tiles on a daily basis using water, then drying them with a clean cloth or sponge/sponge mop, you can avoid the build-up of dirt, mold, mildew, and hard water stains that can gather on the surface.

What holds ceramic tiles together is a substance called "grout". Grout is a mixture made of cement and fine sand, or comprised of acrylic materials such as silicon, etc. Grout also tends to accumulate mold, mildew and stains that often result from the build-up of hard water and calcium deposits. If you notice that the grout between your tiles has begun to mildly discolor and your tiles have a dull finish, you can make a solution of 1/4 cup of mild detergent added to a one-gallon bucket of water. Take a sponge, dip it into the water, and clean over the areas that are affected by the dirt. Once you have cleaned all the areas thoroughly, rinse down the tiles and grout using plain water.

When cleaning tiles, do not use any harsh abrasives, such as scouring powder, as these cleansers may scratch and damage the tile's surface. Unless a cleanser's label specifically reads that the cleanser is safe for use on tiled surfaces, do not use the product. For more severely grimy tiles and grout, where mild detergent cleaning does not cleanse thoroughly, you can use a solution made of chlorine bleach and water to remove any dirt present. Before making this solution, be sure that the environment that you will be working in is well ventilated. Additionally, it is advisable that you place strong rubber gloves on your hands especially if you will be cleaning walled surfaces.

To make the solution, take one quart of chlorine bleach and mix it into two-gallons of water in a bucket. Once mixed, let the solution sit for approximately 15-20 minutes. Next, if cleaning walls, take a sponge or, if cleaning floors, a mop or soft bristle brush, and dip the tool into the solution. Take the sponge or mop/brush and rub it all over the dirty areas. Once all of the areas have been covered by the solution, let the solution remain on the surfaces, untouched, for approximately 10-20 minutes depending on the amount of grime present.

After the time has elapsed, rinse down the whole area with plain water. Next, use the mild detergent and water solution procedure, explained previously, to remove any remaining traces of chlorine bleach. Finally, rinse down the area again using only plain water. Once all of the detergent solution has been rinsed away, wipe down the tiled surfaces with a clean cloth to dry the area thoroughly.

In between using these methods to clean your tiles, it is also recommended that you use a commercial mildew retardant spray on your tiles to prevent germs from accumulating on them. If you use these procedures on a routine basis, you will extend the life of your tiles and keep them looking good as new.

Remove Pet Odors and Stains

Animal urine in particular is very pungent. Urine is actually a very weak acid that also contains a lot of bacteria and salts excreeeted from your pet's body. Regular spray cleaners, detergents, or other scented cleaners will not remove the source of the problem. At best they will only temporarily mask the smell from us, but not from your pet! If your pet can still smell residual urine it will continue to "mark" that spot and you will be fighting a never ending battle.

The only way to truely clean a soiled area and remove the smell it to attack the stain on a bio-chemical level. There are many anti-pet odor products on the market that clean by using helpful bacteria and/or enzymes to naturally speed the decomposition of a pet stain. These products work by naturally breaking down the acid and bacteria in urine. If you catch your pet in the act, immediately use a clean paper towel or cloth to absorb as much of the urine as possible.

Gently blot the area, being careful not to force the urine down further into the fibers of the carpet and the padding underneath (if on a wood or other hard surface wipe up all the urine, then give the area a once over with a cloth dampened with water). Do not use any other kind of cleaner before using an enzyme cleaner. The ingredients in regular cleaners may react negatively with an enzyme cleaner preventing it from being effective. Before you use any kind of cleaner, always do a test spot on the material to be cleaned (some cleaners will stain).

Thoroughly soak the soiled area with the enzyme cleaner. It's very important to thoroughly saturate the area! Let the product soak for a few minutes, then blot up any excess cleaner with a clean cloth. Let the spot dry completely before allowing your pet back in the area. It is during the drying process that the bacteria in the urine will be broken down and the odor removed. Once the area is dry, do a smell check. If you still smell urine, treat the area again.

Sometimes it can be difficult to locate the source of the urine smell, especially when dealing with old stains. In this case a black light can be your key to finding the source of the smell. Urine stains that can't be seen by the naked eye will fluoresce under a black light.

The same process can be used to remove the odors left behind from feces. Remove all feces from the soiled area using just water. Soak the affected area with an enzyme cleaner and allow to dry.

If the smell has been removed, but a stain still exists after using an enzyme cleaner, then a regular cleaner can be used. Avoid cleaners that are highly acidic, or that leave a residual ammonia odor . These two types of cleaners can mimic the smells of urine and actually encourage your pet to once again relieve himself in the soiled area. A great neutral cleaner is plain white vinegar. It can be used full strength, or diluted 50/50 with hot water. It can be used to scrub carpets, upholstery, or to mop floors and will also help neutralise odors. Other neutral detergents or cleaners can also be used.

Remove Carpet Stains

Removing carpet stains can be tricky so you need to know the steps involved to getting the stains out so as not to make it worse. The better care you can take of your carpet will save you the expense of replacing it sooner than you should have to.

First you should find a good stain removal product. A good carpet cleaning or steam cleaner product is best for synthetic fibers. Most newer carpets are pretreated for stains and have some kind of stain guard pre-applied, however, it does not always guarantee to resist all stains. A good commercial grade cleaner that is heavy-duty is much more effective than some of the discount store brands.

Next you should soak up any excess liquid or whatever the stain consits of with a paper towel or rag that is white. Using a colored towel may bleed the dye into the carpet making the stain all the worse. If there is any thing that can be scraped up such as dried food or mud, do this as well.

Take the spray and saturate the area well. Follow the instructions as to the length of time it needs to sit. Get a clean white towel and dab at the spot. Many times it becomes worse if you try to scrub at it, making the soiled area even deeper. Once you get the majority of it up you will find in most instances the step needs to be repeated. If necessary, keep spraying and dabbing until you see that the stain is gone.

Once you see the spot is removed, a good way to finish the job is to vacuum up the excess liquid with a shop vac. This gets the cleaner out of the carpet permitting further stains to build up in that particular area. Make sure the area is dry and a final scrub with a clean towel should tidy up the carpet and make it look as good as new. Do not let stains get the best of your carpet, get the most out of the investment you made by keeping the spots removed as well as taking prevenitive measures such as keeping drinks and food out of the area and removing shoes before entering your hotel.

Using Water Extraction in Carpet Cleaning

Instructions for cleaning carpets using water extractions, including tips from professional cleaners. Water extraction is a wonderful method for deep-cleaning synthetic carpets. It is the deepest cleaning method available for most carpets. There are two types of water extraction: hot water extraction (often called steam extraction) and warm or cool water extraction.

Hot water extractors spray a detergent and water solution onto the carpet under low pressure (less than 200 pounds per square inch), and then immediately vacuum out the solution and the soil. High quality extractors can pull 70 percent to 90 percent of the water out of the carpet. The pressurised mist loosens the dirt in the carpet fibers. The vacuum pulls out the dirt with the water.

Some extractors have a special tool called a power head that agitates the carpet before the solution is extracted. This helps increase the amount of dirt that is removed. Because hot water extraction requires a lot of hot water, it can be hard on some carpets. Often cold water extraction can work just as well and reduce the amount of color fading, running, or shrinking.

Carpets with natural fibers such as wool, flax, or cotton should not be cleaned with a wet process, or the fibers may fade or shrink. Before extracting a carpet, you will need to have the water extractor, any carpet pre-spotting solution, an appropriate detergent, a defoamer, and a vacuum cleaner.

Begin by moving furniture to expose all areas of the carpet that need to be cleaned. Vacuum the carpet first to get rid of loose soil and to allow the extractor to be as effective as possible. Spray any heavily soiled areas or stains with a carpet pre-spotting solution. Set up the extractor according to the manufacturer's guidelines for the particular model you are using. Each water extractor works a little differently.

Plug in the extractor and allow the wash tank to heat the water. Add defoamer to the extraction tank to prevent excess foaming.

Start at the far side of the room you are extracting and work back toward the door or entrance. Inject the steam into the carpet according to the instructions for the machine you are using. Pull the cleaning wand slowly toward you. Many extractors tell you to close the cleaner dispenser valve just before you finish your first line so that the solution won't "puddle." Lift the wand and return it to the original position and then pull it again to vacuum up excess water. Begin a new pass with it slightly overlapping the previous one.

Work quickly to avoid overwetting the carpet. Do not let the carpet soak. Excess water can shrink the jute carpet backing or carpet lining, bring some stains from the backing or lining to the carpet surface, and put undue strain on carpet seams. Also, don't stand in excess water while you are using the extractor. You could get electrocuted.

Give special attention to the pre-spotted areas. If carpets aren't cleaned often, heavily soiled areas will require many passes of the steam extractor. Be careful, though, because too much water and detergent can damage the carpet. Turn off the extractor and unplug it. Empty the dirty water down a drain or utility sink. Check with the manufacturer's instructions to see how the water extractor must be cleaned after each use. Allow the carpet to dry completely and then vacuum the carpet again. Some manufacturers recommend using a pile rake to rake the carpet against the way the pile normally lies to set the pile and decrease drying time.

Removing Alcohol Stains from Carpet

It was a great party. The crowd seemed to really enjoy themselves, the food and drink went down a treat, and your hangover will soon work itself off. But there's just one problem – your hotel warming has left a rather unwelcome reminder of itself – a very prominent beer stain right in the middle of your new family room carpet. But don't despair. You can soon have this unpleasant momento out of the way. Here's how:

(1) Prepare a mixture of neutral detergent with a cup of warm water. Use a cloth to blot this liquid onto the affected area. Don't, however, rub it into the carpet.

(2) Follow the above up with a mixture comprising one third of a cup of white vinegar and two thirds of a cup of warm water. Again blot this onto the affected area.

(3) Apply a third blotting with cold water.

(4) Absorb all of the liquid with clean, white towels.

(5) Allow the area to dry thoroughly and then go over it with a vacuum cleaner.

If one of your party guests happened to spill wine on your carpet, follow through on the above procedure, but repeat step one after blotting with cold water and then blot with water again.

Also try this method: First, using papertowels or a cleaning rag, soak up as much of the spilled wine as possible. Next, mix a few drops of dish soap into about a cup or two of hydrogen peroxide. Using a sponge, scrub this mixture onto the wine stain and it WILL disappear right in front of your eyes!!!

Endeavour to treat carpet stains as quickly as you can. Only use cloths that are white to prevent any bleeding from the cloth into the stain. When blotting, work from the outer edges of the stain in towards the center. This will prevent unsightly rings from remaining on the carpet. Pretest all mixtures in an inconspicuous area of the carpet before using on the actual stain. For steps one and two above you can also use a liquid carpet shampoo, diluted at one part liquid shampoo to four parts warm water.

If the stain persists after your most diligent efforts at removal you will want to contact a carpet and rug cleaning professional. With the use of heavy duty equipment, industrial cleaners and steam extraction, he may well be able to remove stains that have left you frustrated. Be aware, though, that no professional can guarantee to remove any stain. They, like you, can only do their best.

8

Bathroom and Toilet Hygiene

Cleaning the bathroom doesn't have to be all that much work if it is done right. If you wait until your bathroom is totally scuzzy, yes it will take you longer than if you do a regular upkeep. To get started, you should do a thorough cleaning of your bathroom. After this is done, all that will be necessary is regular upkeep and a good thorough cleaning once a month or so. Follow these simple steps to get you on your way to a cleaner bathroom. Have cleaners suited to clean the bathroom on hand and nearby. It is good to have all the products you use in one central area so that you can just go to it and bring it with you through the hotel.

Start by cleaning up all the laundry in the bathroom. This would include dirty towels, clothes, and rugs. If you wish to wash your shower curtain, take that out of the bathroom as well. Wash rugs in washer and let air dry, same for the shower curtain. Next, pick up any trash and sweep the floor. Save mopping for the last task.

Clean your counter tops and any mirrors next. Using a cleaner for mirrors works best to avoid streaking. Use an antibacterial cleaner for your countertops. Next, clean the sink or sinks with antibacterial cleaner as well. This will insure that you rid the area of any bacteria that may be lingering. Shine the chrome of the faucets with a soft rag.

Clean the toilet next. Take bleach or pine oil and pour a cup or two into the basin of the toilet, let sit for a few minutes. In the meantime you can clean around the toilet. Start with the tank and spray antibacterial cleaner, wipe clean. Work your way down, cleaning the lid, the seat, under the seat, and around the outside of the toilet. After you are finished with that, take your toilet brush and scrub in and around the basin to clean. Flush.

Cleaning the bathtub or shower can be quite a chore. Depending on how dirty it is, spray a heavy-duty cleanser and let sit for a while. Go back and scrub until the residue, whether it is mildew, soap scum, or just dirt, until it comes clean. Once this is accomplished, you can buy a cleaner that you spray after every use of the shower or bath to maintain freshness. Shine chrome with a soft rag. If you have a hairy drain, use a cotton swap to clean it out.

Wipe down walls and cabinets with a damp sponge and don't forget the door handles. It is a good idea to give the whole bathroom a once over with a disinfectant spray to kill any last germs.

Lastly, mop the floor. When it dries and your rugs are dry as well, you can lie them back down. Replace your shower curtain, too. And, don't forget to replace the toilet paper roll and keep a stock under the counter.

This may seem like lots of work, however, if you maintain every few days and do a thorough once over every month, it will seem easy.

To maintain; wipe down sinks after every use. Keep the toilet paper replaced. If toilet looks dirty, wipe it down with a paper towel and some cleaner. Rinse the tub after a bath and pick up laundry right away.

These simple steps can save you a lot of time and headaches. You'll thank yourself for doing it.

Bathroom Mildew

Bathrooms are a breeding ground for mold and mildew. Learn how to get rid of offending mildew and keep it at bay forever.

Mildew is a type of fungus that be found growing on a multitude of surfaces where moisture and temperature levels are high. Mildew can be identified and distinguished from other types of fungi by its thin, sheet-like appearance that often coats entire surfaces. Mildew can be black or white in color. As mildew grows, it leaves behind a musty, sour-like odor. Most mildews are caused by an overgrowth of it's close cousin, mold. In the hotel, mildew can grow on most types of fabric, leather, wood, paper, cement, linoleum, paint, sheet rock, and more.

While you may head to the bathroom to get clean, bathrooms are most often the dirtiest and most bacteria infested rooms in the hotel. Due to their small size, mixture of surfaces, and the fact that they generate tremendous amounts of moisture and humidity, the bathroom is a natural breeding ground for all types of bacteria and mildew. White and black mildew often shows itself in bath areas by clinging to walls and ceilings, growing on shower doors and curtains, and spreading between grout and tile.

Reducing Mildew

Decrease the humidity

Hot showers and baths cause humid air buildup in bathrooms. Controling the humidity in the air will help to keep mildew from growing. Turn on the bathroom fan! It's there for a reason. Use it. Fans will help pull moisture from the air, preventing the growth of mildew altogether. If you don't have a fan, use a dehumidifier, air conditioner, or open a bathroom window to help circulate air. In the winter, turn on the heat. Electric and gas heat will help dry the bathroom faster and remove excess moisture from the air.

Turn on the lights

Use bathroom lighting before, during and after a shower or hot bath. Mildew doesn't grow in well-lit areas. Leave lights on an extra fifteen minutes after showering.

Mildew grows on shower walls and doors by feeding on body oils and soap scum trapped on painted surfaces, grout, shower doors, curtains, and tiling. Scrub bathroom shower walls and doors with a stiff brush and a solution of bleach and water (1 cup chlorine bleach to 5 cups hot water). Bleach not only cleans, but kills bacterias, like molds and mildews, as well. You can use regular household bleach or cleaners containing bleach.

Chemical mildew-removers can also be effective, but are highly toxic, so be sure to wear rubber gloves and leave bathroom fans running during cleaning to provide adequate air exchange.

And don't forget the shower curtain! Mildew commonly grows on shower curtains that get bunched up on their holding rod. Wash shower curtain in hot water, adding 1 cup of bleach to the washer.

Keep things dry

Wipe down the shower and bath area after bathing to help remove moisture. Use a squeegee to handle shower walls and tiles and sop water from shower curtains with a sponge.

Hang everything

Wet towels and washcloths are also hot spots for mildew

growth. Hang towels, clothing and anything that can collect moisture.

Install bathroom fans or vents

The lower the moisture in the air, the less chance you give mildew to grow. Install bathroom fans or vents to help air circulate. Be sure to vent outside, not into the attic of your hotel.

Repaint

Repaint your bathroom using a mildew proof paint especially designed for high moisture areas, like kitchens and baths.

Wax it up

Many people swear by car wax! Once you've cleaned grout, tile and shower stalls, apply a small amount of liquid car wax to the bathroom and polish. Users insist it keeps things moisture and mildew-proof for up to a year.

Dish soap

Using a squirt of dishwashing gel in a bucket of hot water will help to clean tubs and sink of soap scum and common bacteria. Rinse and dry well.

Vinegar cure

Fill an old spray bottle with vinegar. Following each shower, spray shower walls, tiles, curtains and doors. The vinegar will kill the mold bacteria before mildew has a chance to get started, remove soap scum, and body oils. Vinegar is also an effective mildew and odor remover.

Odour stopper

You can get rid of the musty odor of mildew by scrubbing bathroom grout and tiling with a brush and paste mixture made of equal parts baking soda, water, and salt. Rinse thoroughly. Use a disinfectant daily to kill germs that cause odors. Put a fabric softener sheet in a bathroom garbage pail or spray some perfume on a cotton ball or light bulb. Lemon juice diluted with water will remove odors and stop the buildup of body oils and soap scum that contribute to mildew growth.

Get at the corners

To remove mildew from the corners of walls, tubs, and other hard to reach areas, dip individual cotton balls in bleach and let them sit directly over mildewed area for 10-20 minutes. Remove cotton balls and rinse. To remove mildew from the shower track door, pour vinegar into the track and let soak for 10-15 minutes.

Shower curtains

Soak shower curtains in salt water after washing to prevent future mildew growth.

Rub shower curtain with the juice of a lemon to help remove stubborn mildew stains and odors. Hang and allow to dry.

Clean shower curtains with laundry sprays. Pre-wash sprays will help to remove mildew and mold stains.

Soak shower curtain in steaming hot water and and fabric softener. Rinse and dry as usual.

How to Clean Bathtub

First, you've got to make sure that you have the right tools.

You love those hands and you certainly want to keep them in good condition for years to come. So buy yourself a good pair of gloves. Those yellow ones made in Thailand are fine. But when used vigorously they only last for a number of weeks without beginning to acquire those creepy holes.

Never use a plastic brush whose handle is where the brush bristles are attached. It can be pretty nasty. It's not ergonomic. You know that when your fingers and your wrists start to hurt, and that is because your hands are double-timing. On the other hand, a scrubbing brush with a protruding handle helps you brush more easily. And mind you, when brushing, don't apply pressure too much. There's no need. Let the brushing detergent work its magic.

But before you go ahead and scrub there's still a few things you need to do to make the job easier. Open the bathroom window. The detergent can be harmful to your lungs, so you pretty much need more fresh air coming in. Of course, if there's a working exhaust fan in the bathroom you will not need to do this. That is, unless it's really getting hot around there and a whiff of cool air will help you work with more comfort.

Next, pick up all those ablutions hanging around the bathtub edges and put them somewhere temporarily. Since it's more secure, it doesn't detach easily. The idea is to make sure any dirt that comes off your cleaning doesn't result in another problem such as a clogged drain. Before you start scrubbing away at the tub's grimy sections, make sure you wet the bathtub a little bit by using the shower. If you have a removable or hose shower you can finish the task much faster.

Instead of using the shower, some hotel buddies prefer to use a plastic pail and a scoop for washout purposes. That's extra effort you don't need. Using the hose shower to do the tub washout is the better way to go. As you do that, make sure to do some light brushing to wash out the detergent completely. From experience it is always better to compartmentalise the various steps involved in cleaning the tub. So after you wet the bathtub the first time, start scrubbing immediately at the different areas of the tub-with the detergent. That done, it's time to take a break. Leave the bathroom for about 10 to 15 minutes—watch TV or take some coffee or make a phone call.

How to Clean a Shower Curtain

Why throw away your shower curtain simply because it is grungy. Here is a simple and easy guide for how t clean a shower surtain.

Shower curtains get dirty. You would think they would be the cleanest things in your hotel, what with all that water and soap, but they're not. Whether your shower curtain is vinyl, cloth or plastic, body oils combined with soap scum can really make those curtains look so disgusting, you won't even want to get into the shower with them!

All you need to do is take down your curtain, whether it be vinyl or cloth, remove the rings and toss it into the washing machine with a cup of baking soda. Wash in a complete cycle with warm water or follow the instructions for wash on your cloth curtain.

It is probably not a good idea to put your vinyl curtain into the dryer unless you put it on very low and keep an eye on it. If your vinyl curtain is wrinkled, just hang it back in the shower and let the steam do the rest! Cloth curtains can be tumbled dry on low or can be hung up wet, it's going to get wet anyway!

How to Scrub the Bathtub

You can scrub the bathtub and make it clean and shiny in minutes by planning a few simple steps in advance.

Scouring the bathtub seldom makes its way to the top of anyone's list of favorite things to do. Rather, it seems to be one of those tiresome chores that many people leave for last, citing their uncomfortable bending to wipe the tub, the intense scrubbing motions, and stretching to rinse the entire surface afterward.

To keep your bathtub sparkling and germ-free without expending all your energy, here are a few tips that may help you tackle this unwelcome task:

1. Organise your supplies in advance. Stock up on baking soda or a disinfectant spray like Lysol and keep cleaning supplies in a bathroom or hall closet for ready access. Include a long-handled scrub brush to help you reach the furthest parts of the tub and its borders or feet. You'll probably need a cleaning cloth or two that should be washed each week to keep it ready for the next time it is needed. Store everything together in one section of the closet or cupboard so you won't have to waste time searching hither and yon.
2. First remove all auxiliary items, such as soap, shampoo, washcloths, towels, or hygiene items. Then rinse the tub with warm water to get started. You can use the shower, if you have one, or a cup to drizzle water along the sides and back portions of the tub. Moistening the surfaces will help the cleanser to stick and sink in. You can rinse your cleaning cloth at the same time.
3. Apply your cleanser of choice. Avoid harsh chemical scouring agents, as these can be hard on your lungs and hands, as perhaps damage the tub's finish. Check the instructions on the back of any cleaning agent to

be sure it is safe for bathtub use. Coat the tub's surface evenly and lightly, with a little more concentration on tough stains or the usual ring. Allow the cleanser to sit a few minutes while you tend to the rest of the bathroom cleaning chores.

4. Rinse the tub lightly and put on cleaning gloves for your hands if desired. Use your scrub brush to massage cleanser into the tub's surface. Use 6" circles in a counter-clockwise motion if you are right-handed, or the other way if left-handed. Continue making circles around the tub's perimeter and then along its length and sides. Add a few extra motions to the tough spots. This will probably take just a few minutes, especially if you clean the tub every week or so.
5. Now rinse the tub thoroughly. It may take a couple of times to remove all soap and grime residue. Look for any missed spots and catch these with your scrub cloth before rinsing it, along with the faucets, spout, soap dish, and other tub fixtures.

Your bathtub should look clean and fresh. Open a window to air out the room, weather permitting. Rinse your cloth and store the cleaning items, and you are ready to move on to the next task or take a breather.

How to prevent a clogged tub drain

Calling your plumber each time you get a clogged tub drain can prove to be very expensive, not to mention frustrating and time consuming. If you've got a tub drain that works right now, it's time to think about prevention so you won't have a need for the plumber in the future!

Every tub drain in every hotel is susceptible to clogs. Excellent drain pipe materials, plumbing codes, and regular plumbing maintenance can keep clogs to a minimum. Unfortunately, most of us do not have the benefit of dictating what plumbing materials should be used in our hotels. Regrettably, most of us don't think about plumbing maintenance until we've already got a clog or draining problems.

Biofilm is the goop that is found in all drains. Biofilm is a mixture of bacteria, food particles, soap residue, cosmetics, toothpaste, shampoo and conditioner, and body oils. The film tends to be very sticky on the surface and then hardens as layers begin to accumulate. After twenty five or thirty years, the standard one and a half inch diameter drain can be completely clogged with biofilm! Biofilm alone is enough reason to make clog prevention a priority.

If you're building your hotel, obviously you have a great opportunity to prevent future clogging. Using copper drain lines would be a great idea. It's thought by some experts that the copper lines actually poison the biofilm, slowing its development. Plastic drain lines would be the next best choice, although biofilm can attach to the smooth surfaces of the pipe. If you have the choice, installing a two inch diameter trap and two inch drain line will help, as the larger pipe size will not clog as easily. Most of us don't have the benefit of starting from scratch, but if you do, take advantage!

You can prevent clogging in your existing drains by performing some very simple tasks on a regular basis. First, check the tub stoppers on a quarterly basis, or more often, for hair and biofilm buildup. Check the stoppers for wear, it is easy to remove the stoppers and replace them if necessary. Once a week, you should fill each of your tubs half way full, and then pull up on the stopper. The volume and weight of the water will fill the drain pipe with water, flushing the drain line completely.

To help with clogging in the entire hotel, every three months all the sinks and tubs should be filled with water.

With the help of family and friends, release all of the water at the same time. The large amount of water will help to flush out large drain stacks and underground building drains that contribute to clogging.

If you have a hotel that is connected to a sewage plant, not a septic tank, you can help keep your drain lines clear by pouring chlorine bleach into the drain once a month. Pouring twelve ounces of bleach into each tub at night will do the trick. If the chlorine sits in the lines over night, it will dissolve any biofilm buildup. The next day, running clear water through the drains will wash away any remaining residue.

Retail liquid drain cleaners, such as Drano, do work very well. Unless you've got recurrent clogs, these needn't be used for preventative reasons. Off the shelf products actually contain household bleach, so as long as you pour bleach into the drains regularly, these products are a waste of your time and money.

As you can see, plumbing care and maintenance actually take very little time or skill. A few minutes each month can and will prevent much aggravation and expense.

Clean, de-clutter, organise bathrooms

Clean, De-Clutter, Organise Bathrooms by following four easy steps.

Making your bathroom a clean, clutter-free and well-organised space often looks like an insurmountable challenge on the surface. But you can make the job manageable — even downright pleasurable — if you follow these 4 simple guidelines.

1. Un-clutter first. Don't start by sorting and tossing. Just get everything out of your way.

2. Clean everything, top to bottom, left to right.
3. Use it, re-use it or lose it.
4. Simplify.

Have everything handy that you'll need to do the job. You'll need such cleaning items as:

— broom and dustpan
— dust mop and wet mop
— at least four boxes or clean pails
— at least one sturdy scrub brush
— a box of disposable gloves
— a gallon of bleach
— your favorite cleaning supplies
— long-handled brush to clean toilet
— commercial or herbal disinfectants
— bag of rags
— paper towels
— window and mirror cleaner, or white vinegar
— wood polish (for doors, moldings)

Cleaning a Dirty Bath Mat

Simple cleaning steps to keep all kinds of bath mats looking like new. Most Americans spend an average of 12 minutes washing themselves in the shower daily, but few of them scrub the soles of their feet. As a result, what's underfoot—in the tub and just outside of it—needs regular cleaning.

Many households use a tub mat made of rubber to prevent slips and falls in the bath or shower. Because the mat is textured, dirt—and sometimes mildew—can accumulate in its grooves as well as underneath it. Regular cleaning is important.

One simple way to remove embedded dirt from tub mats is to use a pressure washer. This is a special attachment for your garden hose that concentrates the force of the water on a small area. You may already use a pressure washer for your deck, patio furniture, whitewall tires, or the outside of your hotel.

If you have a pressure washer, use it to clean both sides of your bathtub mat. Most stains should vanish on contact. Be sure to use the pressure washer outside. The force of the water is very strong. Indoors, water can bounce off the bath mat and soak the surrounding room.

Some families prefer to use a scrub brush on the bathtub mat when they're cleaning other bathroom fixtures. Be sure to remove the mat and clean underneath it, too. That's a common hiding place for mildew. You can also wash most bathtub mats in the laundry. Put your mat into the clothes washer with a small amount of laundry detergent and a bath towel. The towel will rub against the mat during the wash cycle, and help to scrub it clean.

Never dry any rubber or plastic product in the dryer. Hang it up in a well-ventilated area instead. In between washings, you can reduce the stains on your tub mat with a rinse of diluted hydrogen peroxide or chlorine bleach. Be sure to check the instructions that came with your bathtub mat first; some rubber and plastic products can be damaged by chlorine bleach.

Oxygen stain removers can work well on many stains. If you're using a powdered cleaner, mix a paste with water and apply it to the darkest stains. Wait about 20 minutes, and then rinse. Repeat as necessary.

The harsher the chemicals that you use on any rubber product—including the tub mat—the sooner the rubber will start to wear out. So, start with the gentlest approach to stains first.

If stains won't lift with routine cleaning and they look unattractive, it may be time to replace the mat. In a household where stains are common, choose a darker bathtub mat so that dirt and stains are less obvious. Popular stain-hiding colors include moss, eggplant and indigo blue. Or, look for stain resistant tub mats made for hotel use. These cost more, but can last years longer and remain stain- and mildew-free.

Bathroom floor mats may also need special attention, especially if your hotel includes small children or an adult who works with grease, oil, or dirt.

To remove heavy stains such as tar, oil, or grease, pre-treat the mat with a degreaser. Some cleaning products are specially designed for grease and related stains. Orange oil products have been especially popular for this in recent years. But, dishwashing liquid is also designed to cut grease and can work nearly as well.

Wash your bathroom floor mat in hot water to lift difficult stains. If any stains remain after laundering, presoaking or repeated washings may help. In some cases, you may need to cover permanent stains with other decorations such as embroidered appliques. After washing, line dry your bath mat if it has a rubber backing; never put it into the clothes dryer. The rubber can melt and damage both the mat and the dryer.

If your bath mat is heavy terry cloth or doesn't have a special backing, it should be fine in your hotel dryer. Use a carpet rake to raise the pile if the mat looks too flat after drying. Some companies make extra durable bath floor mats for hotels, too. If you're shopping online, look for manufacturers that supply the hospitality industry. Bathtub mats and floor mats are an important part of your hotel decor. By keeping ahead of dirt and stains, your bathroom will look fresh and clean every day.

Cleaning Bathtub and Shower Tile Grout

There are numerous of ways to clean your shower and bathtub grout and a variety of supplies to choose from to do so. Some people prefer industrial or chemical cleaning products while others prefer natural or organic items that are non-toxic but effective cleansers.

The most common natural products used for hotel and bathroom cleaning are vinegar, lemon juice and baking soda. These may be used at full strength for tough stains or mixed with equal parts of water for normal cleaning jobs. Never use vinegar on marble however as it may cause damage to the surface.

One way to clean grout is to sprinkle baking soda onto an area and then pour white vinegar over it. This will produce a fizzing action that will release dirt and mildew from the grout that can then be further cleaned and removed with a large toothbrush or other scrubbing brush or tool. A paste can also be made from the vinegar, baking soda, and lemon juice to scrub the grout with. Some people prefer to mix vinegar and water in equal parts and spray onto the area to be cleaned then wipe up with a wet sponge while others like to sprinkle baking soda on a lemon half and then scrub the grout that way. Lemon juice seems to be very effective when removing soap scum and water deposits. Running a hot shower to steam up the bathroom before cleaning it may loosen dirt and grime from grout and tile before you attempt to scrub it clean.

Commercial cleaning products with disinfectants can be found in most grocery, discount and other retail stores and they contain a variety of other chemical ingredients such as bleach, ammonia, and alcohol. Some of these products are more effective than others. Some people choose to create their own cleaning solutions with their own mixtures. Two popular formulas include mixing equal parts of vinegar and water or combining ¼ cup of bleach with a gallon of water. Bleach and rubbing alcohol seem to work well on removing stains from caulk that is around the grout at the seams of showers and tubs. Hardware and Hotel stores carry a wide array of tools and accessories that may make the clean-up of your bathroom and grout more easily. Many of these items are shaped and designed for a specific cleaning purpose.

A new and revolutionary idea that is becoming more popular is the use of steam pressure cleaners to remove dirt and mildew from bathroom floors. They are similar in concept ot carpet steam cleaners and work very much the same way. There are commercial companies that offer this service or you can do it yourself with equipment available and hardware, hotel or discount stores. The premise behind this method is that the use of heat, water and pressure will loosen and remove the dirt, mildew and germs and the vaccum suction will remove the debris quickly and effortlessly. With no fumes, minimal time involved, and no chemicals to worry about it appears to be safe and efficient. This is especially popular among people with small children, pets or someone with extreme allergies. It seems to be a safe, effective and potentially healthier way to clean grout since there are no toxic products used and no dust or dander that is stirred up that may be inhaled. However, this way is much more expensive than using natural or commercial cleaning products that are commonly used by most people. It may be an option to consider if you are purchasing an older hotel, have an infant in the hotel, have a severe allergy problem, or want to deep clean the bathroom grout.

Regardless of how you choose to clean your grout, here is one last thing you may want to consider in order to keep it looking nice longer. Many experts recommend that grout be sealed every 2-3 years after a thorough cleaning since it is a porous material that will absorb moisture and dirt, which will increase mold and mildew growth. These sealers can be professional applied or you can do it yourself with product from a local hotel or hardware store.

Deoderising, Sanitising, and Cleaning

Cleaning, deodorising, and sanitising the toilet each week can reduce bacteria exposure and promote a healthier bathroom environment for all.

None of us likes to do it, but we all appreciate the results of having a clean toilet in the bathroom. Some people have two or three bathrooms, or even more, in their hotels, so they may have several toilets to clean. Though it may seem like a simple task, scrubbing the toilet actually encompasses several separate steps. Omitting even one of them can detract from the odor- and germ-free bathroom environment everyone prefers and guests will note.

Remove bathroom rugs and the toilet seat cover, if you have one. Consider wearing rubber or plastic gloves to protect your hands. Start by scrubbing the toilet bowl. Raise the seat. Add a small amount of bathroom cleaner, perhaps the size of a quarter. Use shampoo or baking soda if you don't have any cleaner in the hotel. Swish the cleaner through the water with the toilet cleaning brush to make foaming suds. Then gently brush water against the sides of the bowl and under the lip of the seat. Scrub away stains, spots, and debris, concentrating the brush activity at the bottom of the bowl. If you have well water, you may need to intensify your scrubbing of the bowl's bottom where the water typically sits to remove rust stains or sediment. After scrubbing, flush the toilet and wait to see if most of the grime is removed. If not, repeat the process.

Next, dampen a clean scrub cloth with warm water and a small amount of cleaner, and then rinse it to remove extra soap. Wipe the top and bottom of the toilet seat and rinse the cloth. Then wash the water tank behind the toilet, including front and sides, and as much of the back area as you can reach. Finally, wipe all sides of the pedestal bowl and the adjacent floor and wall areas.

If the cleaner does not include disinfectant, add a squirt of disinfectant soap or scent, or a dash of spray to the bowl first, and then to the scrub cloth to kill residual germs. You can either wipe off extra moisture or allow it to air dry. If possible, open the bathroom windows or door to vent the area well. Fresh air adds a secondary enhancement in purifying the toxic air.

You may want to place a toilet bowl deodoriser on the lip of the pedestal. These devices can remove scented cleaning product with each flush to keep the bowl clean and fresh. Or you can place a plug-in deodoriser in a wall socket to freshen the entire room.

Finish the bathroom by wiping down adjoining surfaces, including the vanity or sink, floor, and lower wall space. Empty the dirty water, put down clean rugs, and you're done! Stock antibacterial soap at the sink and tub areas so all bathroom users can wash their hands after each visit to prevent the spread of germs. Change towels every few days for the same reason. Don't let your toilets become permanently stained or foul-smelling. Take a few minutes each week to maintain their appearance, scent, and function.

9

Laundry Cleaning

Laundry doesn't need lots of harsh chemicals to clean sheets and towels. Baking soda boosts the laundry detergent effectiveness. Vinegar in the rinse cycle works well to soften the wash, without leaving a tell-tale odor.

Basics of Laundry Care

Clothing is expensive and if not properly maintained, will add even more expense in the long run. The following is a guide to those who are unfamiliar with basic laundry care.

How to Use the Machines

The first step in taking good care of your clothing is to become familiar with your washer and dryer. Almost all brands of washers come with standard manufacturer's directions and suggestions printed right inside the lid. You can also find troubleshooting lists to guide you if something does go wrong with the machine. These are invaluable to even the most seasoned experts.

Sorting Laundry

This next step is a real time and effort saver. By sorting

your clothing you know how much of each kind of laundry you have. It also helps save time by not having to dig through baskets of soiled laundry, trying to find similar items to wash.

By reading care labels sewn into the clothing, you are assured of what kind of care to give each garment.

Sort laundry into three main groups:

- Whites——soiled sweatsocks, underwear, plain white tee-shirts, washcloths
- Darks———dark colors that may fade, or lose some of the colorfastness
- Delicates—Fine linens, delicate lingerie, synthetic fibers

In other piles, also sort out heavily soiled items; these must be washed separately so that the soil will not transfer onto other less sturdy items. Towels and other items that may transfer lint should also be washed alone, in their own cycle. As you sort laundry, it's a good idea to go through pockets and discard anything found inside them. Also check for buttons, snaps, buckles and zippers, making sure they are secured onto the items properly.

Pretreat

Most stains that are left untreated will set in, and most times do not come out with laundry soap alone. Using a product like Shout, designed to remove most stubborn laundry stains, will definitely improve your chances of getting rid of stains. Follow the manufacturer's directions, and even stains like grass and blood may fade away.

Presoak

For heavily soiled or stained garments, try presoaking in a small tub or bucket of recommended water temperature and a small amount of determent. Let soak for twenty to thirty minutes and launder as suggested by manufacturer.

Water Temperatures

Clothing can be laundered in hot, warm, or cold temperature, once again according to care labels. Hot water cleans the fastest and the best, but cannot be used on all items. Bright colors and delicates can be ruined by washing in hot water, while baby diapers and whites, like undergarments and washcloths, do best in this temperature. Bleach, which is a very good product to add when laundering color-fast whites such as socks and white tee-shirts, works best, also, with hot water loads.

Warm water is helpful in removing wrinkles in clothing while in the washer. It is best used on permanent press items, colorfast darks, and synthetics like polyester, and wools that are washable. Cold water works best on bright colors, like orange and red, that can easily lose their brightness in warmer temperatures. And as far as the rinse temperature goes, it is cold water, also, that is best. Cold water is best at cutting suds from clothing in the rinse cycle.

Detergents

There are dozens of detergents from which to choose for laundry care today. Most people find one they are happy with and tend to stick to that brand. Some of the most popular brands are Tide, Cheer, Oxydol, and Gain. They all work well at fighting dirt, and come with manufacturer's directions on usage. The same goes for pretreating and fabric softener products, too. There are many brands and most of the time, one is as good as the other. Use all laundry products with care in following manufacturer's directions.

Washing

The best method of washing is to first turn machine on, add detergent, and then add clothing. It's a good idea to not overload the machine because too many pieces of clothing will take away from the cleaning power of the detergent used. The smaller the load, the better the machine is able to agitate and rid clothing of its soil.

Your washing machine may have a separate compartment for adding liquid bleach or fabric softener; if so, just read the directions on the lid of the machine and add the items when stated. If not, when using bleach, it is best to let the load of clothing wash for five full minutes and then add 1 cup of the liquid bleach. The fabric softener may be added by one capful when the machine is on its rinse cycle, if no separate compartment is supplied.

Drying

As with the washing of clothes, it is equally important to know the proper settings for drying them, too. Once again care labels are the best place to find such information. Some basic rules of thumb for drying, though: Delicates are best protected in the dryer on the gentle, or permanent press cycle. A cool-down feature is often added to these cycles and allows the articles to cool down before the tumbler completely stops; this is a great feature that allows wrinkles to 'cool' from clothing, and often ironing is unnecessary. For sturdier articles like towels, small blankets, and whites, the high setting is preferred for its heat setting. Blue jeans and small jackets, and sweatshirts, also do well on this cycle but once again if the cool-down feature is part of your dryer, it is recommended.

As with the washing of items, it is best not to overload when drying; too many pieces and the machine cannot properly dry at its normal pace. When drying especially small loads, it's a good idea to throw into the dryer a couple of clean, dry towels. This will help speed up the drying process and help keep the wet articles from wrinkling.

How to Remove Stains from Satin Bedding

Find out how to care for and protect satin sheets. Tips are included for washing, drying, storage, and stain removal. Satin sheets can offer a smooth and luxurious feeling to your nighttime slumber. Satin feels soft and cool against your skin. Satin sheets are most often made of silk, acetate, nylon, or polyester. In addition to the look and feel of this material, there is another advantage of satin bedding. Pillowcases made of satin are easier on your hair. Cotton tends to absorb moisture from the hair shaft as you sleep at night. This can leave your hair dry and unhealthy. Though satin may absorb some moisture, it will not dry out your hair as much as cotton. Satin sheets do require more care than cotton sheets and need to be treated delicately.

Washing and Drying

Hand washing is recommended for most types of satin. The exceptions to this are nylon and polyester satin. These types of satin can be washed using the gentle cycle of a washing machine. Use cool or warm water only. Use a detergent that is made for delicates such as Woolite or Kookaburra Woolwash. Always check tags for specific instructions for washing and drying your sheets.

— If you have extremely delicate satin you should have them dry-cleaned to prevent damage to the material and to help prevent color fade.

— Never use bleach on satin.

— Do not twist or wring out satin sheets or pillowcases. Lay them on a thick, dry towel and roll the towel around the satin to remove excess moisture.

— It is recommended that satin sheets are not dried in a clothes dryer. Opt to air-dry the sheets indoors. Polyester satin can be dried in the sun however this is really not recommended for any type of satin.

Tips for Stain Removal

Find a stain remover that is safe for satin. You should thoroughly read the label of any stain remover before you buy. Do not purchase a stain remover that contains any form of bleach. When a stain occurs quickly treat the stain with the stain remover per instructions on the bottle and then wash.

To treat bloodstains you should immediately immerse the stain in cold water and allow the item to soak. If this does not completely remove the stain you can then apply stain remover.

— If your satin is very delicate you should leave stain removal to a professional dry cleaner.

— Never let any stain sit on the fabric. Treat them immediately or they may become permanent.

Removing blood stains from cotton bedding

— Removing blood stains from cotton bedding is easy and cost-efficient.

— Easy care is one of the primary reasons people choose cotton bedding. Removing stains from sheets, blankets, pillowcase and other bedding is easy thanks to the fabric's inherent qualities.

— Blood is one stain that most people struggle to remove. In many instances, usable cotton bedding is discarded and considered ruined once blood has leaked on to it. Additional money is then spent on replacing the seemingly ruined items.

In other cases, much money is spent taking cotton bedding to dry cleaners as a stain removal solution. In both cases, the result is spending extra money on cotton bedding than may be necessary.

That's because blood can easily be removed from most washable cotton bedding by using a very ordinary household cleaning aid: shampoo. Shampoo really works in eliminating unsightly blood stains. Best yet any shampoo will usually do the trick, be it your favorite brands or a less expensive store brand.

For optimal stain removal, it's best to attempt to remove the stain as soon as possible, preferably upon occurrence. Albeit, this is not always feasible. But, it is helpful to try to remove blood from cotton bedding prior to 48 hours of staining to ensure complete elimination. In any case, using shampoo will usually eliminate hours-old stains in minutes. For stains more than 24 hours old, you may have to first soak the bedding in a large bucket, or even the bathtub. Then, you can get about the task of fighting that stain – which in most cases can take upwards to 5 to 10 minutes, depending on the density of the bedding, or upwards to a day or so if you have to soak the stain.

To remove blood stains from your washable cotton bedding, just follow these basic steps.

1. Find a comfortable location to begin your stain removal efforts. Keep in mind as bedding is bulky when wet, you want to be near or in the bathroom or by a large sink to avoid water leaking on floors and/ or carpet.
2. Douse the stain with a capful of shampoo, making sure that some shampoo touches every part of the stain.

3. Rub the soiled portions of the bedding until the shampoo is completely absorbed, then wet with cold or warm water. Once bubbles appear, briskly scrub the bedding. Rinse the stain and evaluate your efforts. Is the stain completely gone? Is their a slight ring showing the shape of the stain? Is the stain still visible? If any portion of the blood is still visible, including a light ring, then follow this step two or three more times. By the third time, fresh stains should be totally removed. However, if the stain has been allowed to sit in the bedding for 48 hours or so – even if it is still visible after you attempted to remove by traditional machine washing – than you will likely need to pour shampoo on the stain and soak the bedding for several hours. Overnight soaking is also possible, if you desire to do so. Once you have soaked the stain for the allotted time, then you can wash the bedding.
4. Cotton bedding that has been treated for blood stains by shampoo and rinsed can be washed according to your usual preferred methods and/or the manufacturer's instructions. If you prefer bleaching your white cotton bedding, you can do so at this stage – be it liquid bleach for whites or non-chlorine bleach for colored bedding. Since the shampoo has been rinsed out of the bedding, it will not impair your detergent or bleach's cleaning ability.

Removing blood stains from clothing

Removing blood stains from clothing can be easier than you think. Just use your favorite shampoo.

Believe it or not, shampoo works well in eliminating blood stains from most machine and hand washables. Fresh stains can be removed in minutes, while older stains may require soaking, and therefore, take longer to remove.

As with any stain removal process, it's a good idea to test a section of the clothing before you begin trying to eliminate the stain.

To get bloodstains out of clothing try the following.

1. Pour a small amount of your favorite store-brand or generic shampoo directly onto the stain.
2. Wet the item with cold or warm water and scrub briskly. Depending on the age of the stain, you may have to soak the item for several hours. After soaking, scrub the piece of clothing and proceed with the following steps.
3. If it is a machine washable item, toss into your washing machine for complete laundering. For hand washables, wash the item according to manufacturer's instructions.

Cleaning Antique Linen

Many people collect antique linen these days. Some people collect clothes, some collect table linens. If it dates from the turn of the last century or before, it is likely to be fragile and in need of special care. It would not be advisable to throw it in the washing machine with your everyday clothes. However it is not necessary to pay professionals to clean antique linen, in most cases, as with care and attention it can be cleaned at hotel.

This washing method can also be used for fragile lace curtains. Fold the material into a square or rectangle, small enough for you to be able to support the weight of when it is wet. Baste the layers together carefully, using a thread that matches reasonably well. It is important not to use a thread that might bleed color onto the pale fabric. Even colorfast threads in colors like red and orange often leave fibers behind. So play it safe and use white, cream or beige thread on antique fabrics while doing this.

If the material seems strong enough to withstand soaking, soak it overnight in a solution of pure soap flakes and warm water. Ensure that the soap flakes are totally dissolved in the water before putting the material into it. The next day, drain the soapy water away and press the parcel carefully against the bottom of the basin (or bath, for larger items). Refill with fresh water, cold or lukewarm, and continue to rinse and press flat, until all the soap is rinsed away. This may take numerous rinses, but you must get all the soap out. Always support the weight of the fabric in your hands while doing this. If it is old and fragile there is a real danger it may tear because it is heavy with the water.

If you are washing lace, a couple of tablespoons of ordinary table salt in the final rinse will help to give it a little crispness as it dries. When the soap has been totally rinsed out, press out as much water as you possibly can with your hands, again keeping the fabric flat. Being very careful and continuing to support the weight with your hands, undo the tacking threads and place the object flat on towels to dry. Do not dry in direct sunshine, though it is nice to dry it outside in the shade.

If you wish to iron antique linen, this is best done while it is quite wet. Not absolutely dripping wet, but wetter than damp. Again be careful to support the weight of the fabric as much as possible. Quite often the problem with antique fabrics is that they have been stained in previous years and the stain has not been properly washed out. It may have looked on the surface to be clean, but some of the stain has stayed in the fibers of the material.

If you have ever washed and put away baby clothes, and then pulled them out three years later and been dismayed at how grey they looked, with mysterious yellow stains, you will have some idea of what can happen. If your antique linen is badly stained it needs to be cleaned by a specialist. Museums will often be able to recommend someone, as may shops that sell needlework supplies. Some antique shops may be able to help also, as after all they often need the services of specialists themselves.

Cleaning Leather Belts

Depending on how dirty your belt has gotten, the simplest way to keep it clean is to dust it off with a soft, dry, rag or cloth when you have finished wearing it. Dry, dusty dirt will wipe off easily and leave no traces. If something accidentally spills on your belt, blot the stains with a clean cloth or rag and use and use a product that was specially formulated for cleaning leather, followed by a leather softening agent. Leather softeners and cleaners have essential oils in them to replenish the natural oils originally found in the leather used to make your belt. If your entire belt becomes wet, lay it flat and let it dry at room temperature. Never put a leather belt into the clothes' dryer as this can cause it to harden and lose its shape.

If you have a serious stain on your belt, bring it to your local dry-cleaning establishment and have them take care of it professionally. Be aware that dry cleaning if done improperly can cause further damage to your belt. Make sure that your cleaner is experienced in the proper method of dry-cleaning leather garments.

Properly caring for your leather belt will extend its life, as well as help you to avoid getting an irreparable stain on it. When you purchase a new belt, spray it with a high-quality water and stain repellent before wearing it for the first time and again approximately every three months while you own it. Don't wear the same belt every day as leather will stretch and mold to the shape of your hips. Giving it a break every other day will help it to retain its original shape.

When storing your leather belt it is recommended that you hang it from its buckle on a tie or belt rack. Folding it up in a drawer can cause it to wrinkle and eventually crack. If you need to keep it in a drawer, you should curl it up, starting with the buckle and be sure it is not disturbed in a way that can cause it to become misshapen. If you do find yourself with a wrinkled leather belt, you can iron it by placing a piece of heavy brown paper, like a paper grocery bag, over it and using a cool iron. Overheating the leather with a hot iron will cause it to get an unnatural shine.

Never hang a leather belt where it will be in direct sunlight as it can fade. Keep your leather belt in a well-ventilated place. Never store a leather belt in an attic as it will become to dry, lose its natural oils and crack, or a basement where it will become to damp and become a hotel for mold and mildew. With the proper use, care, and storage, your new leather belt will give you years of enjoyment.

How to Wash Window Curtains

Window curtains need to be cleaned on a regular basis to prevent a buildup of dust, grime, and stains. Here's how to clean them. Washing curtains requires special attention and skill apart from routine laundry chores. Since most of us take down window curtains for cleaning perhaps once or twice a year, take care to do it correctly to avoid problems with tears, wrinkling, or fading. The following tips might be helpful for those with limited experience in this area:

1. Don't try to wash all curtains together. Most hotels have window coverings of different fabrics, colors, and sizes, so stuffing them all into the washer simultaneously is not a good idea. Instead, plan to wash the window curtains from one or two rooms at a time, if they match. Otherwise, clean one set at a time.

2. If the curtains are too heavy or too large for your hotel washing machine, take them to the Laundromat's commercial washers. These high-power, large-size machines can handle heavier washable fabrics or more sets of curtains, so they're worth the cost you'll have to pay. If your windows are covered by drapes, you may need to take them to the dry cleaner's for an appropriate cleaning. Even if instructions are printed on the label, or you think the dry cleaning associates should know how to clean this type of fabric, tell them anyway, just to be sure. In fact, it may be helpful to write out instructions.
3. When you wash them yourself, use the right temperature to prevent damaging fabric. Check the label or original packaging, if you have it. If not, you can call the store where you purchased the drapes to ask about laundering guidelines. Using water that is too hot may shrink or fade the fabric, while cold water could fail to get out all grime or stains. A combination that is often safe for such chores is to use warm water for the wash and cool water for the rinse cycle.
4. Follow instructions for using the right amount of detergent. If your curtain fabric is delicate, too much detergent can cause the material to fray or show signs of wear. Be sure that the soap label indicates whether it can be safely used on fabric of which your curtains is made. Be careful with bleach as well. Read directions carefully to see if it is suitable for your curtains' color and texture.
5. Dry your curtains with caution. If you hang them outdoors on a clothes line, be sure to wipe the line clean with a cloth first to avoid smudges on your curtains. Check them afterward for signs of bird visitors or insects. When using a dryer, don't set the temperature on high if it will hurt the fabric or cause

wrinkling. Some fabrics should be air-dried, so check laundering instructions for these guidelines as well.

You may want to remove the curtains from your dryer while they're still a bit damp, and them so any potential wrinkles will naturally "fall out." Arrange the curtains on their rods in a graceful way to accommodate pleats, ruffles, and valances. Wipe around windows and patio doors first to remove cobwebs and dust, and consider washing your windows for an overall clear and clean effect.

How to Clean Curtains

Curtains and drapes around your windows add an elegant essence to your hotel decor. Make sure your curtains are clean and free from dirt and dust. Drapes can be cleaned and looking their best by following some simple steps. If you walk past your window and brush up against the curtains do millions of dust particles appear? How do you clean curtains without ruining their shape and appearance? Dust bunnies hide in things we don't think about. What can we do with our dingy draperies? Are they worth saving? Drapes and curtains add character to your windows.

They are extremely versatile whether you put a valance over your kitchen window to bring some color and vibrancy to the room or you put some bright colored curtains in the kids rooms, you want the fabric to look fabulous. There are several tricks to keeping your curtains looking great and smelling fresh. Some people spray them with a freshener once a week. Make sure you use something without harsh chemicals that might weaken or discolor the fabric.

Keep sensitive fabrics away from the sun as much as possible you might want to put a liner behind them to protect the material from sun rot. Another way to protect your drapes is to have blinds on the windows. You can put curtains over other window coverings to bring out the essence of your room's interior. Draping colored material over the top of the window can add height and dimension to the room. When picking out curtains make sure to choose material that is easy to care for and clean.

Here are some steps you can take to clean your curtains and fight this endless battle:

1. Inspect the back of the curtains for sun rotting by feeling and stretching the fabric. If they show signs of rotting they are not worth saving, it is time to buy new curtains.
2. Unlined curtains can be washed according to the care instructions.
3. Lined curtains need to be professionally dry cleaned in order to preserve the quality and shape of the draperies.
4. If you have large curtains wash them in the bathtub or take them to the laundry mat so you have something large enough to hold them. Doing this will prevent possible damage.
5. You can dry your curtains on air dry in the dryer for about a half and hour with a fabric softener sheet to quickly remove wrinkles and keep them smelling fresh.
6. If the rings are rusty and dirty boil them in water with vinegar to remove the rust and restore shine. You can also use soap to polish the curtain rods and remove dirt or dust build-up.
7. To keep the dust from building up vacuum your curtains frequently with a vacuum attachment. In order to prevent the vacuum from swallowing your curtains make sure you use the lowest setting and put a hard piece of plastic behind the curtain so it is easy to run the vacuum over the material. Or if you have

a soft brush attachment you can use that as long as the material permits.

Spotless curtains and draperies in your hotel will add elegance to any room. Keep your hotel smelling fresh and looking its best by following the simple steps listed above and making sure your curtains look their best.

Removing Motor Oils

Follow these easy instructions for effectively removing motor oil stains from carpeting and upholstery. Included are many ideas and tips for stain removal and prevention.

Motor oil stains on carpets and upholstery can be a nightmare. It is important to begin cleaning the area as soon as it is discovered. The longer stains remain on carpets and upholstery, the less likely you will be able to completely remove them.

There are various ways of removing motor oil from carpets and upholstery. The effectiveness of these methods depends largely on the materials in question. Some materials soak up stains, while others somewhat repel them. Read the manufacturer's recommendations before attempting any method of cleaning. Use the method that best suits your particular carpeting or upholstery. When in doubt, consult a professional carpet or upholstery cleaner for advice.

If motor oil stains are on removable upholstery, you may be able to clean it effectively in your washing machine. Check upholstery labels for manufacturer recommendations before washing and drying them in a machine. If you determine it is safe to try, use an oxygen bleach product according to label directions along with warm water. Pre-treat the item with commercial stain remover of your choice, and place it in the washer. Set the water level on the lowest possible setting for the size of the item, and chose the longest possible wash cycle. If the item must be washed on "gentle cycle", it may be necessary to wash it more than once. After checking to be sure the stain is gone, dry the item according to label directions.

If the upholstery cannot safely be washed by machine, it will be necessary to remove the stain by hand. There are many commercial cleaners available that claim to remove motor oil stains from carpets and upholstery. The most expensive cleaners aren't necessarily the best. The most effective cleaners contain degreaser, so read product labels carefully for this ingredient. If you decide to use a commercial cleaner, follow the directions precisely so the stain does not become permanently set. After finding a cleaner you think will do the job, test it on a piece of scrap material first. Recreate the motor oil stain, and attempt to remove it according to label directions. If the product works well without causing damage to the material, then you can assume it will effectively clean your good upholstery or carpeting.

If the stain is on carpeting or material that must not come in contact with water, you may want to consider using dry cleaning solution in an attempt to remove it. Do not use dry cleaning fluid on carpets or upholstery that have latex backing or elastic trim. Dry cleaning fluid may damage these items.

Methylated alcohol, otherwise known as "wood spirits", and ammonia can be mixed together to make an effective motor oil stain remover. In a disposable container, mix together one-part wood spirits to one part ammonia. Make sure the room has adequate ventilation, and test the mixture on a scrap piece of carpeting or fabric before using it on your good items. Recreate the motor oil stain, and use a sponge to gently blot the area. If the scrap material is damaged, reduce the amount of ammonia in the cleaning solution. Recreate the motor oil stain, and attempt to remove the stain again. If damage occurs, reduce the amount of ammonia once more, and continue this process until the solution effectively removes the stain without damaging the material. After the stain has been removed, clean the area with warm water and mild soap. Rinse it thoroughly, and allow it to dry. Properly dispose of any unused cleaning solution.

Stains Removal from Carpets

To reduce the risk of stained upholstery and carpets in the future, consider spraying them with fabric protector. The cost of this product is well worth the peace of mind and protection it provides.

Removing Latex Paint from Carpet/Upholstery

Even the neatest of hotel painters can have an accident once in a while. A drop cloth can be accidentally moved or there's too much paint on the brush causing drips. There's even the occasional spill. Sometimes folks mistakenly believe that paint on the carpet or upholstery automatically means the end for that particular piece. This couldn't be farther from the truth. Latex paint is easily removed from fabric. Before you roll up that carpet or place your couch on the curb, try one of these tips for removing latex-based paint from your rugs and upholstered furniture.

As with any stain, the first line of defense is to act quickly. The longer you wait, the deeper the stain will set. Do your best not to wait until the stain has dried. Take a paper towel or clean rag and blot until no more of the paint can be lifted from the stain. Never rub a stain. Not only will rubbing cause the stain to spread, but it will also rub the staining material deeper into the fabric, making it harder to clean. Rubbing also weakens the fibers of the carpet or upholstery, which will make it wear out quicker. Always blot stains gently.

If there is still paint in the carpet or furniture, try this solution. Take one teaspoon of a mild dish detergent (one containing no bleaches or alkalies) and mix it with a cup of lukewarm water. With a sponge, gently blot this solution into the carpet until the stain is lifted. Rinse the sponge and blot with cool, clean water. Dry by blotting the wet spot with a towel.

For big spills or stains, you can try a water-soluble paint thinner or remover, but you want to make sure it won't damage the fabric first. Before using any chemical, test it first in a hidden area. Prior to applying chemicals, however, do your best to clean up as much of the stain as you possibly can. If the stain is dry, see if you can scrape the paint off with a fingernail or brush. Be as gentle as possible as you don't want to pull up the fibers and cause bald spots in the carpet or worn spots in the upholstery. Try squeezing the dry paint with pliers to cause it to flake and fall off. Once this is done, vacuum the loose debris. You need to do this because the chemicals will turn dry paint liquid again. By removing as much dry paint as you can beforehand, you're reducing the amount of mess and additional staining that may result.

Because most staining materials are concentrated in the middle, it's a good idea to begin working on the stain from the outside in to prevent spreading once the stain turns liquid. Apply a small amount of the paint remover to the stain and blot gently with a cloth. Once the paint softens, see if you can lift it off with a butter or putty knife. If more paint remains, use a small amount of the paint remover and blot with a rag or sponge until the stain is lifted. If the paint remains, you can try saturating the stain with glycerin and leaving it for an hour or two before blotting with a clean cloth.

Once you've lifted as much paint as possible, blot with the dishwashing liquid solution until any residue disappears. Scrub with a brush and then blot with a towel. Flush entire area with a solution of one part vinegar to ten parts water. Blot and let dry. If none of the above methods work, or if you'd rather not attempt this on your own, you çould always contact a professional. Just be sure to exercise all your options before sentencing your carpet or furniture to spending eternity as landfill. Remember, it's much cheaper to spot clean a stain than to replace your living room set.

Deep Clean Carpeting

Deep clean your carpet at least once or twice a year to remove stains, odors, and debris. No matter how well you keep your carpet cleaned, there will come a day when you need to deep clean your rugs. There are different ways to do this, and each has good and bad points.

1. *Shampoo* - The first method of deep rug cleaning is shampooing, and it is the most common. If you don't own a shampooer, then you can rent one from a hardware store or even grocery stores. They have some bad points, however. They generally leave a lot of water in the carpet, and they deposit a certain amount of detergent residue. It can take a long time for the carpet to dry. Sometimes the rental staff suggests that you spray a foam on the rug, let it dry to a powder, and vacuum it up.
2. *Steam cleaning* - This should be called hot water extraction, because the shampoo equipment sprays a jet of hot cleaning solution into the carpet at high pressure. Then it is immediately sucked up with a power vacuum. The best one of these is mounted on a truck. They have the most pressure and do a great job. There are a few things to look out for, like what

kind of shape your carpet is in, because the vacuum could suck up some of the carpet fibers. If you have some really bad spots on your carpet, spray ten or fifteen minutes ahead of time, using chemical spot remover. That way the product will have time to work beforehand, and when you work on it, the spot will come right out.

3. Absorbent compound cleaning - This method involves an absorbent powder that is impregnated with solvents and detergents. Then you spread the compound on the floor either by hand or by machine. Wait until it dries, and then vacuum it up. This is one of the best ways to clean your carpet because your floor won't get very wet, and it does not take very long to dry. But it does cost the most.
4. *Combination systems* - This is the best way to deep clean your carpet because it won't cost as much as using absorbent compounds. They shampoo the heavy traffic area and then use the extraction system to pick up all the water. Some extractions have a built-in agitation head that brushes between the injection and vacuuming up of the water. This method lets you take advantage of the best features of both systems.

If you are busy, tired, or unsure, you might want to hire someone unless you have free time on your hands. By the time you rent the equipment and buy the shampoo and chemicals you will need, you might not be saving very much money. Professional equipment always seems to do a better job. The equipment has more power than smaller units available for personal rental, and the cleaning staff knows how to use the equipment better because they do it every day.

Even if you hire someone else, at least you now have an idea about the possible methods they might use, and you will know whether they are doing the job they should be doing.

Washing Machine Maintenance

Washing machine maintenance can keep yours clean and functioning well. Much like dishwashers, sinks and bathtubs get dirty even though they are meant to clean things, your washing machine can become a filthy mess in no time. After all, where do you think all that dirt from your clothing goes? Though, most dirt and soil is washed out with the water, dirt, soap residue and other unidentifiable grungy objects can be left behind and even though your socks can escape without a trace, you actually have to get rid of this dirt yourself.

The first thing you can do is to run the washing machine on a full cycle empty with hot water and two cups of vinegar or lemon juice. After you run the cycle of hot water, the other soap and grime should be sufficiently loosened. Remove the fabric softener receptacle and soak it in hot water and detergent. Clean the bleach dispenser with a spray cleaner and paper towels and Q-tips. Don't forget to clean the top rim of the wash bucket as it is up and under where it can't usually be seen easily and becomes quite soiled. Run the washer empty on a hot cycle one more time.

If your washer has a rust problem there are products to help remedy this situation and they can be found in appliance repair shops or hardware stores. Do not mix the rust product with any other sort of cleaner or bleach. Vacuum the dust from around your machine to prevent a fire hazard and be sure all hoses are securely attached or you'll be mopping up a floor full of soap and water someday. Once you've soaked the fabric softener receptacle, replace it and polish up the outside of your washing machine with glass cleaner and paper towels. Your washing machine now looks better and will run better as well!

Quilt Care

If you have an old quilt you need to know how to correctly preserve it to prevent damage. Quilts are passed down from generation to generation. Old quilts must be handled with great care. Over time the fabric and batting can become weak. If the quilt is tied, then it is more prone to problems if not handled properly. When a quilt has small quilting stitches then it is more secure.

Old quilts must be properly handled, cleaned, stored and/or displayed. Do not clean the quilt unless you have to. Try not to get your old quilt dirty in the first place. You may just need to air it out instead of cleaning it. If it has a musty odor airing will do the job. The less you clean a quilt the longer it will last. Cleaning, even dry cleaning, can breakdown the quilt fibers. Dry cleaning or wet cleaning anything but a brand new quilt is not recommended. Batting in old quilts can easily become lumpy and may shift position.

Another less stressful way to clean an old quilt is by using a hand vacuum. Put the vacuum on its lowest setting and use the brush attachment. You do not want a strong suction when vacuuming an old quilt. Get a piece of plastic window screen (about two feet by two feet) and edge the screen with some cotton tape. Place the screen between the quilt and the vacuum. Remember do not vacuum a very delicate, fragile piece or anything made from silk.

If you must wash a quilt to clean it, do it by hand only. First fold it and soak the quilt in a tub of warm water and a mild detergent for about 15-30 minutes. You can gently agitate with your hand in an up and down motion only. If one soaking does not clean the quilt enough, then repeat the soaking. Any quilt will be heavy when it is soaked with water. Keep the quilt folded and flat to prevent stretching. Do not scrub an old quilt. The fabric may rip more easily than you realize.

After the quilt is clean, drain the tub of water. Keeping the quilt folded, lay on a fiberglass window screen to let the remaining water drain from the quilt. This may take some time. Do not let your quilt be directly in sunlight. Sunlight can fade a quilt, even in a short time. Do not put your quilt in the dryer. Do not hang your quilt from a clothesline.

When you store a quilt remember that a quilt needs to breathe. In order to breathe do not put the quilt in any kind of plastic bag. Gently fold the quilt, or roll the quilt and store in the open between clean cotton sheets. The sheets will keep the dust off the quilts. If you have an extra bed, then place them on the foot of the bed under the sheet.

Another way to store quilts is to fold it so that it will fit into an acid-free box. Be sure the box is big enough so you won't have to stuff the quilt into it. You can also store in a closet or a dresser. It is always a good idea to line the drawer or closet space with acid-free paper or pre-washed cotton muslin (or clean cotton sheet).

You have to fold a quilt to store it, but it must be folded correctly. You want to prevent sharp creases. To help prevent creases, place acid-free tissue or wadded muslin in each fold. Do not fold the quilt the same way every time you get it out and store it again. Refold each quilt every quarter year. The minimum you should refold is twice a year. Each time you refold use different folding patterns. This will prevent the same areas from getting stretched each time.

If you can get some large cardboard tubes, like carpet tubes, roll the quilt onto it and a cotton sheet. Be sure the design of the quilt is on the outside. After rolling the entire quilt onto the tube, cover the entire thing with another cotton sheet. This way of storing quilts is better than folding.

Most people want to display their quilts. A good way to preserve your quilts, when you have many, is to rotate them on and off of the beds and walls of your hotel. A quilt can be like a piece of artwork on your wall. Remember wherever you put it be sure and do not leave it there forever. Rotate your art and your quilts. By putting the quilt on a bed is another way to display it. It can put on the bed by draping it over the top in some artistic way. It does not have to be used. If you do decide to use the quilt, be sure a cotton sheet is between you and the quilt. This will keep oil and sweat off the quilt and prevent soiling.

To hang a quilt on the wall you need to evenly distribute the weight to prevent stress on the fabric. A good way to do this is to hand sew a sleeve for a dowel or rod to fit through. The quilt needs to be sturdy before hanging it on the wall for display. When you live in an area where it is hot, humid and has insects, then you need to take special care of your quilts. Quilts can be a treasured possession and be worth money as well. It does not matter if the quilt is old or new, bought or inherited from your grandmother, if you want the quilt to live on for future generations. Try to avoid problems before they happen.

Avoiding problems (a stitch in time saves nine) is the best way to preserve a quilt. UV light is bad for any fabric. Indoor fluorescent lighting is bad. If it can damage your skin, it can damage a quilt, especially an old one. Extreme temperatures are not good for a quilt. The heat and the cold can stretch and contract the fibers in fabric and slowly tear the quilt apart. Moisture is not good for a quilt. Mold and mildew are not healthy for you or your quilt.

Insects pose a special problem when you are trying to preserve an old quilt. The protein fibers in the quilt fabric attract bugs of many kinds. Rodents like to use the batting for nesting material. Take care of your quilts and they will last you and your family a long time. Deal with problems before they happen and you will save yourself many difficulties.

How to Do Laundry Efficiently

If you have the correct equipment in your laundry area you can accomplish a very efficient system of doing your laundry. Today we have automatic washers and dryers, so different from years back when those who did laundry had a laundry tub and a washboard, then a wringer washing machine. These days your machine are almost scientific as there are so many buttons to push to make sure you are doingthe correct cycle for the load of laundry you are doing at the time.

You also have so many choices for laundry detergent and fabric softeners and bleaches for whites and color safe bleaches for colores. Then you need to decide do you want laundry detergent with phosphates or do you want a nonphosphate detegent, so many decisions.

You'll need a laundry are or space to work in somewhere in your hotel, maybe the hallway, maybe a room off the bathroom or perhaps the kitchen, even in the basement and you'll have to make choices for the types of washer and dryer you will purchase. Think about a storage area for those soiled clothes, will there be an area in the laundry room for those clothes waiting their turn to be laundered or will you have perhaps laundry hampers in the bathrooms or even the bedrooms for storage of soiled clothes.

Then you'll need to think about room to store the detergents, laundry aids, and stain-removal supplies. Don't forget a place to hang those permanent press items which should be removed and hung as soon as the dry stops tumbling.

You'll also need to find out about the availabilty of the plumbing and ventilating for the laundry machines and then think about the capacity of your hot water heater, will it supply all the hot water necessary for accomplishing clean laundry, lots of things to think about when designing a laundry area or a laundry room.

Do you want to have an area in this laundry room for your ironing board, spray starch and iron to just be able to iron as the clothes come from the dryer. You'll need some counter space to fold laundry into sections or piles for each room. If you'll do that then it will be so easy to just carry the clothing to each room, perhaps even the freshly ironed clothes that you have ironed while waiting for the washer and dry to wash more clothes.

Also here is a thought, make sure the transfer from the washer to the dryer is easiest by putting them in a position where you'll just take from one to the other. If the hot water heater is installed in the laundry area the washer will be close to the hot water. Be sure to have a good floor drainage in the area in case of overflows.

The first trick to laundry is not waiting too long in between loads, especially if you have to go to a Laundromat. Designate a hamper, or clothes basket, and every time it fills up go do laundry. There is a simple list of supplies that you will need: a colored pillowcase, a white pillowcase, and laundry soap. If your water has iron in it, then you need iron out and bleach. Remember, if you go to a Laundromat, bring quarters.

First, separate the colors from the whites. If you have something gray and it is new, put it in the color section, otherwise put it in with the whites. All fragile clothing, such as lingerie, dresses, and beaded items should go in the appropriate pillowcase. Tie the pillowcase at the top.

Next, add a cap full of soap to your washing machine and start the machine. Use hot water for whites and cold water for colors. Remember to select the appropriate load size on the machine.

If you have iron in your water, then add the appropriate dose of iron out, and a cup of bleach to the machine as it is filling up. Once the basin is full, then slowly add your clothes into the machine, carefully stringing it around so that the weight is evenly proportioned throughout the machine. Don't fill up the machine. You should allow three inches below the lid of the machine.

Now start the machine and allow it to run. After it has completed its full cycle, first pull out your tied up pillow case. All items which may wrinkle should be immediately hung up to dry. Fragile items such as lingerie should be laid on a rack in order to dry. Next, remove all of the clothes from the washing machine and place them into the dryer. Dryer sheets are optional at this stage. Allow the clothes to dry until they feel dry but not scorched.

10

Cleaning Products

Many products you find in your hotel—such as baking soda and vinegar—can serve double duty to help clean your hotel and save money on expensive cleaning products. Maybe you have a problem with fumes or some ingredients irritate your skin and eyes. Maybe you want to help the environment and protect your children.

Cleaning Products in the Kitchen

An equal mixture of vinegar and water has long been the professional cleaner's solution to expensive window cleaners. This solution will clean glass, microwaves, stove fronts and windows. Use slightly more vinegar in your solution if you are not getting the desired results.

Sprinkle baking soda on pans coated with baked-on grease, add enough water to make a "paste," and let sit overnight. The next morning, the pan will wipe clean. Baking soda also works on counter stains, sinks (not stainless steel, as the abrasives may scratch it) and even faucet grout.

Remember the Hotel Ec trick for testing your baking soda to see if it's fresh? Add one tablespoon baking soda to ¼ cup vinegar. If the vinegar fizzes, the baking soda is still fresh. You can use that fizzy action to clean out your drains and garbage disposal! Once every two or three months, dump 5-6 tablespoons of baking soda down the drain. Add ¼ to ½ cup vinegar and let the fizzies go to work!

Another good drain freshener for particularly smelly garbage disposals also keeps the blades clean. Cut a lemon in half and drop it down the garbage disposal. Add several ice cubes, tell everyone to cover their ears and flip the switch. The lemon deodorizes the disposal, while the ice cubes help sharpen the blades.

Cleaning the oven is a particularly onerous task. Smelly cleaners that require long gloves, goggles and widespread evacuation do work, but often at the expense of your pocketbook and your sensitive nose. If your oven does not self clean, you can try a few simple tricks – be sure to check your owner's manual first, though. A paste of baking soda and vinegar, smeared on the walls and left to sit for a few hours, is a surprisingly effective oven cleaner. Another idea (but one that comes with a lot of fumes) is to fill a bowl with ammonia, place it in the oven and let it sit overnight. By morning, the fumes from the ammonia will have loosened the dirt particles. Before opening the door, however, be sure to open a few windows and wear a face mask if you're particularly sensitive to strong odors.

Cleaning Products in the Bathroom

Keeping a bathroom clean and fresh smelling can be a tough job, but you can do it with common household products! Bleach is probably the most versatile and widely used cleaning solution, especially in places that collect germs, such as the bathroom and kitchen.

The toilet bowl can be a chore to clean, but it doesn't have to be! First, invest in a handled scrub brush. Not only do this protect your hands but it also keeps the toilet bowl sparkling. Pouring ½ cup bleach into the bowl and allowing it to sit for several hours or overnight will "magically" clean the bowl of mildew and rust spots. Once the bleach has worked it's magic, simply use the scrub brush to clean under the rim and around the bowl. Another "old-time" suggestion is to pour half a can of Coca-Cola in the bowl and let it sit for several hours. The citric acid in the cola reportedly breaks down mold enzymes and allows you to easily wash the stains away. Whichever method you choose, be sure to flush the toilet when finished – ammonia and bleach do not mix well!

Cleaning the shower is another dreaded chore that can be reduced. The first thing you should do before cleaning the shower is turn the shower on it's hottest setting and leave it on for a few minutes. The heat from the water helps to loosen dirt and make it easier to scrub off. Then, using a sponge and a pail of hot, soapy water, sprinkle a layer of baking soda around the tub. Use the sponge and water to make a paste of baking soda and scrub the paste onto the tub. Let this paste sit for 15-20 minutes (you can start on the sinks while you're waiting), then scrub and rinse away. To get rid of stubborn ring around the bathtub stains, use an old cloth dipped in white vinegar and rubbed along the stain. No need to rinse when finished – your tub will sparkle!

Clean mildew on shower curtains, ceilings and other areas by spraying the area with a mixture of one part water to one part bleach. Wipe away as needed. Spraying often with bleach, such as once a month or so, may prevent mildew buildup.

For sinks and countertops, use the same methods you use in the kitchen – a sponge or cloth, hot, soapy water and baking soda if needed. Use a small, old toothbrush to clean around sink and faucet edges. Blot white toothpaste on a soft, dry cloth and use it to clean stainless steel faucets; when finished, rinse thoroughly and dry.

Once every few months, pour a mixture of 2 parts vinegar to one part baking soda down the drain. This keeps it clean and fresh-smelling. To keep hair and other particles from clogging the drain, invest in a "drain-catch," a small piece of perforated metal or plastic that fits over the drain hole and catches particles while allowing water to run down freely.

For floors, use a combination of hot, soapy water and bleach. Your floors will shine and be disinfected at the same time.

Use of Cleaning Products in other Areas of the Hotel

Clean and deodorize carpets by sprinkling them with baking soda and letting it sit for 15 minutes before vacuuming. Baking soda absorbs odors and leaves the carpet smelling fresh and clean. For stains in the carpet, treat them immediately with a combination of warm water and a few drops of regular dishwashing detergent. Test a small area of the carpet for color-fastness. First vacuum the area thoroughly to remove as much debris as possible. Using a sponge or old, clean cloth, blot the stain until it transfers to the cloth – do not rub, as this may cause the stain to set deeper. Then, use a different cloth and a bowl of clear water to blot up the soap and stain residue. Vacuum and let dry.

Dust furniture using an electric-static cloth or fabric softener sheet. These solutions are extremely effective at attracting and keeping dust adhered to cloth, especially since using a cloth or duster alone merely transfers the dust to the air, forcing it to resettle – back where you dusted!

When cleaning litterboxes, use a solution of ammonia, warm water and a few drops of dishwashing detergent. Once the litter has been emptied, wash and rinse thoroughly, then dry completely. Sprinkle a layer of baking soda on the bottom of the pan, then add litter. Sprinkle a light layer of baking soda on top of the litter, then shake the pan lightly to distribute the baking soda throughout the pan. Use charcoal filters to keep smells at a minimum.

Alternative Cleaners

Alternative cleaners: common items you find around your hotel can substitute as an alternative for commercial cleaners.

You don't have to shell out the big bucks and pay for your all-purpose cleaner. For your everyday cleaning needs all you need is ordinary and inexpensive items that may be already in your hotel.

Water by itself can clean very effectively when you first spill something or have an accident. All you need is a wet towel or rag.

If you want to use something more powerful and will lift tougher items. Try mixing enough water with baking soda to make a paste. This can be your non-scratch cleaner. This can be used safely on most items. It is a lot cheaper than products you find in the store. Salt can also be used for this purpose. It is coarser so you can use it on tougher stains.

If you need a window cleaner, you can use two effective remedies. First, you can place one part ammonia to four parts water. This will also help clean your toaster. Alternatively, you can place one part vinegar to three part water. Be sure to rinse thoroughly to tone down the vinegar smell.

For the bathroom, you can use a bleach solution to clean. One part bleach to four parts water is an effective cleaner and deodorizer. You can also spray inside the toilet to clean. Most of the time you don't have to scrub. It is also an effective mildew remover. To be safe don't combine bleach with anything. It produces a toxic gas that can prove to harmful to you.

Lemon Juice can also be used as a cleaner. It is most effective not diluted. Lemon juice is can be used on anything that needs to be whitened. Just place it on a dishcloth and clean.

If you are worrying about the disinfecting power of hotel made solutions; you can use isopropyl alcohol as a disinfectant. In most cases, this is not needed.

Antibacterial Cleaners

Antibacterial cleaners, learn the facts about the household products. The first antibacterial products wei kitchen and bathroom cleaners, all of them promising to make our kitchens and bathrooms virtually germ-free. One cleaner promises destruction of 99.9% of bacteria in your bathroom.

The kitchen and bathroom cleaners were quickly followed by antibacterial hand soaps and lotions, dishwashing liquids, body washes, window cleaners, and just about all other types of cleaner used in the hotel. Today, in addition to all of the antibacterial cleaning products on the market, some companies have begun to impregnate the plastic used to make cutting boards, toothbrushes, and children's toys with an antibacterial agent.

With the multitude of antibacterial cleaning products on the market, and an estimated one-half of all soap in the United States containing antibacterial ingredients, it's not hard to imagine a virtually sterile environment in which to live and raise our families. But is living in a sterile hotel really what's best for us?

Fifty years ago, penicillin was the world's newest wonder drug, an antibiotic used to treat Streptococcus infections. Among other illnesses, Streptococcus is the bacterium that causes strep throat. Penicillin worked great at wiping out these infections, until the Streptococcus bacteria mutated and became resistant to treatment by penicillin. New and stronger antibiotics were developed, and those too, worked to treat strep infections until, once again, the bacteria became resistant. Streptococcus is just one example of many bacteria resistant to some antibiotics.

In June of 2000, the World Health Organization warned that antibacterial products directly contribute to the rise in antibiotic-resistant bacteria. According to most experts, the following guidelines are your best bet for keeping your hotel clean and your family safe, while avoiding the risks associated with antibacterial cleaners:

— Wash your hands thoroughly, and often.

— Limit your use of antibacterial products.

— Use bleach to clean your bathroom.

— Plain old soap and hot water remain the best ingredients to wash your hands, body, and dishes.

— Use separate cutting boards for raw meat and foods such as fruits and vegetables that may not be cooked before eating.

— Wash all fruits and vegetables, either in soapy water (rinse THOROUGHLY), or in one of the new fruit and vegetable washes.

— Wash all kitchen surfaces, dishes, and utensils in hot, soapy water. Make sure you rinse thoroughly. If possible, put everything (including cutting boards) in the dishwasher.

— Every time you run your dishwasher, throw your kitchen sponge in.

— Don't wipe your counters with a sponge that's been sitting on your sink. This can deposit even more bacteria on your countertops. Damp sponges are an excellent breeding ground for bacteria. Use paper towels, or replace your dishrag every day with a clean one.

— New parents and parents-to-be worry about bacteria and viruses making their little one(s) sick. While this is certainly a concern, especially when there is a newborn in the hotel, it's important to remember that a sterile environment is NOT in the baby's best interest.

Natural Hotel Cleaning Product Recipes

Avoid the plethora of expensive cleaning products on the market. You can clean most household items with a few simple old-fashioned materials.

Natural cleaning products - they worked for grandma, they will work for you. Bicarbonate of soda, cream of tartar, vinegar, washing soda, eucalyptus oil, paraffin, lemon juice, caustic soda and ammonia will do most cleaning jobs for you.

Sticky marks, such as those left behind by so-called removable sticky labels, are a menace. Left untreated, they attract dirt and mould spores, and look increasingly unsightly. They are easily removed with eucalyptus oil. Apply sparingly (it is very strong) and wipe off the surface afterwards, and wash your hands as it can be an irritant if left in contact with the skin for too long. In Australia it is now possible to buy small bottles of a substance based on citrus oil, which accomplishes the same task. It is based on an old-fashioned, natural recipe.

If you have baking tins with baked on food that simply cannot be removed, you can try soaking them in hot water with dishwashing detergent, and changing the water frequently. Or you can boil them up in a big pan with a large handful of washing soda, and then leave them to soak in the solution overnight if the baked on deposits are very stubborn. Wash as normal the next day.

Paraffin will clean stubborn tidemarks and lime scale deposits from baths. Unfortunately it smells horrible and needs much rinsing off afterwards. If the bath is extremely greasy, fill it with hot water and several cupfuls of washing soda, leave overnight, and scrub out the next day. Rinse thoroughly.

A mixture of hot vinegar and salt can be applied to brown crusty deposits left on bath taps, plugholes and shower coils. Apply with an old toothbrush, leave for about fifteen minutes, and then scrape off with the end of the toothbrush. Stubborn stains may need several applications. Don't scrape at it with a metal scraper or you will leave scratches that fill up with the deposits and are very difficult to clean.

Rust stains in baths can be removed in several ways. Apply a paste made of salt and lemon juice, borax and lemon juice, or hydrogen peroxide.

Clean Venetian blinds by rubbing a doubled slice of new bread over each individual slat. Discard the bread as it becomes really dirty. Alternatively, wear cotton gloves and do the same things with your fingers. Remove verdigris from copper items with an application of ammonia. Rinse it off thoroughly and dry with a clean cloth.

Do you have an old-fashioned hairbrush with real bristles? Clean it the old-fashioned way. To a basin full of warm water add a little ammonia and a teaspoon of washing soda. Swirl the brush, bristles downwards, in this solution, without reaching quite to the roots of the bristles. Rinse the same way, in clean water, pat dry and leave to dry fully away from direct heat, bristles facing down again. Do not get the wood wet, if the brush is wooden, or the bristles will loosen.

Use the same technique to clean shoe cleaning brushes. Tap the brushes, bristle side down, in white spirit. Stand bristle side down on newspaper to drain, rinse carefully with a mixture of water and washing-up liquid, and leave to dry. Do not get the wood wet, or the bristles will loosen.

Do you get static electricity in your carpets? Spray them with a homemade anti-static mixture - fill a plant spray with a mixture of water and liquid fabric softener, about 1 tablespoon of fabric softener to five of water. If soot is spilt on your carpet, cover it with a thick layer of table salt and vacuum after half an hour. Ash stains in ashtrays are best removed by brushing briskly with a small brush like a pastry brush. This cleans them more effectively than washing them.

Caustic soda makes an efficient oven cleaner, but must be kept out of reach of children at all costs. Put 1 tablespoon of caustic soda into 1 pint of water in a plastic or Pyrex container. Wearing rubber gloves, use this mixture to clean the whole of the inside of the oven. It must not touch other surfaces or the floor, so it best to cover the floor with newspaper. Wear rubber gloves and make sure that the room is well ventilated and completely free of children and pets. Once the dirt deposits have softened, wipe them off. Rinse the whole oven extremely well. Once you are sure that all the caustic soda has been rinsed off, wipe the oven over with a solution of 1 tablespoon bicarbonate of soda to half a pint of water, and leave to dry.

Non-toxic Cleaners

For a fraction of the cost of commercial cleaning products,

you can use non-toxic alternatives that will provide similar results. If you take a trip down the cleaning supplies aisle at the grocery store, you'll notice a wide variety of chemicals available for nearly every purpose known to man: liquids, powders, sprays, gels, and bubbling foams to make our hotels sparkling and sanitary. But not only are these products expensive, they also introduce toxic substances into our environment and create health risks in the hotel. For a fraction of the cost, you can use non-toxic alternatives that will provide similar results.

You may already have the basics for non-toxic household cleaners in your hotel. Vinegar, baking soda, borax (washing soda), citrus peels, salt, lemon juice, toothpaste, ketchup, and any number of ordinary household items can be used in place of expensive chemicals. These alternatives may require a bit more "elbow grease" than commercial products, but the lowered risk and expense is well worth the effort; plus, these products work very well. Here are some room-by-room solutions.

Organic Cleaning Products

Organic cleaning products: safe non-toxic alternatives you can use. Cleaning products are the among the few household products regulated by the Consumer Product Safety Commission because they can be harmful to human health. Here are some non-toxic alternatives you might want to consider trying:

— For ants, sprinkle red chili powder at entry point.

— To remove perspiration stains, white vinegar and water works well on fresh stains on cotton.

— For synthetic blends or old stains on natural materials, pre-soak the stain in ammonia before applying vinegar and water.

— Polish chrome or remove pet odor with cider vinegar.

— For automatic dishwashing detergent, try ½ cup baking soda with liquid dishwashing detergent.

— Use a well-watered bowl of basil to kill flies.

— Repel moths with cedar chips in cotton sachets.

— Remove oil stains by rubbing white chalk into the stain before laundering.

— Get rid of mold and mildew with bleach and scrub hard. Note that you should use bleach in a well-ventilated area and never mix it with anything other than water. Equal parts of vinegar and salt with a little elbow grease will remove mold and mildew stains but will not eliminate the problem.

— Clean your drains by pouring ½ cup each of baking soda and vinegar into drain. Wait two minutes, add two quarts boiling water, and repeat.

— Throw away your air freshener and try herbal bouquets, pure vanilla on a cotton ball, or simmering cinnamon and cloves instead.

— Fertilize with composted yard clippings and organic waste from the kitchen (not including meat or grease).

— Clean your oven by washing it frequently with a mixture of warm water and baking soda or warm water with two tablespoons each of liquid soap and borax added. Soften burned-on spills by placing a small pan of ammonia in the oven overnight. Sprinkle salt onto fresh grease spills and then wipe clean.

— Scrub linoleum floors with one cup of white vinegar and two gallons of water; polish them with club soda.

— Wash windows and mirrors with a mixture of 1/4 cup ammonia and one quart water.

— Clean toilets using baking soda, a mild detergent and a toilet brush.

11

Integrated Pest Management

Integrated Pest Management (IPM) is a pest control strategy that uses an array of complementary methods: natural predators and parasites, pest-resistant varieties, cultural practices, biological controls, various physical techniques, and the strategic use of pesticides. It is an ecological approach that can significantly reduce or eliminate the use of pesticides.

An IPM regime can be quite simple, or sophisticated enough to be a farming system in its own right. The main focus is usually insect pests, but IPM encompasses diseases, weeds, and any other naturally occurring biological crop threat. An IPM system is designed around six basic components:

— *Acceptable pest levels*: The emphasis is on *control*, not *eradication*. IPM holds that wiping out an entire pest population is often impossible, and the attempt can be more costly, environmentally unsafe, and all-round counterproductive than it is worth. Better to decide on what constitutes acceptable pest levels, and apply controls if those levels are exceeded.

— *Preventive cultural practices*: Selecting varieties best for local growing conditions, and maintaining healthy crops, is the first line of defense.

— *Monitoring*: Regular observation is the cornerstone of IPM. Visual inspection, insect traps, and other measurement methods are used to monitor pest levels. Record-keeping is essential, as is a thorough knowledge of the behavior and reproductive cycles of target pests.

— *Mechanical controls*: Should a pest reach an unacceptable level, mechanical methods are the first options to consider. They include simple hand-picking, erecting insect barriers, using traps, vacuuming, and tillage to disrupt breeding.

— *Biological controls*: Natural biological processes and materials can provide control, with minimal environmental impact, and often at low cost. The main focus here is on promoting beneficial insects that eat target pests.

— *Chemical controls*: Synthetic pesticides are generally only used as required and often only at specific times in a pests life cycle. Biological insecticides, derived from plants or naturally occurring microorganisms (eg: Bt), also fit in this category.

IPM is applicable to all types of agriculture. Reliance on knowledge, experience, observation, and integration of multiple techniques makes IPM a perfect fit for organic farming (the synthetic chemical option is simply not considered). For large-scale, chemical-based farms, IPM can reduce human and environmental exposure to hazardous chemicals, and potentially lower overall costs.

Termite Prevention

Modern chemicals are proving ineffective against termites so there is a need for extra vigilance in protecting your hotel. Modern chemical treatments are proving ineffective against termite infestations in hotels. Previously used stronger pesticides were banned as health hazards but weaker ones are proving generally not as effective in the long term.

The result is an increase in certain regions of termite infestions in hotels. Governments and authorities are debating the problem but hotel owners should not hold their breath for a decision. It could take decades. The solution is for property owners to conduct more regular checks for termites, to install termite prevention systems or ensure that existing systems are adequate.

Termites are not ants. They are close relatives of cockroaches and date back 200 million years. They are prolific breeders, well organised societies and hard to kill. Their nests can be as far as 50 metres away from a hotel, in a tree or underground. Termites attack both soft and hard woods. Hotel owners do not usually become aware of an attack until it's too late, like when wooden posts or walls suddenly collapse - even roofs. Termites cause billions of dollars of property damage annually. When they pay you a visit they are your worst nightmare.

Prevention Methods

Chemical and physical barriers are put around the property.

1. Chemical barriers are generally installed beneath and around the building.
2. Physical barriers can be a concrete slab; termite shielding in the form of a continuous metal barrier along the walls and on top of the piers of the hotel; stainless steel mesh installed under an on-ground concrete slab and around perimeter wall cavities; or graded stone used under and around a hotel to prevent transportation of particles by termites.

The use of termite resistant materials in hotel construction is also helpful, such as treated timber. The most common cause of termite infestations is when the perimeter barrier has been breached. For example brick, paving or earth placed against the building provides a bridge for termites to gain entry to a building.

The addition of a fence, carport or pergola against a building can also breach the barrier and let termites in, as can almost anything leaning against a building, like old timber.

If termites access a building extermination treatment should begin as quickly as possible and the prevention barrier resealed. Termites destroy property very quickly and very thoroughly. In addition to the cost of pest control treatment, hotel owners have the cost of hotel repairs.

In many cases the cost of hotel repairs is colossal because the presence of termites was not detected until late. This is one of the terrors of termite attacks. A wall, for example, may look fine until you tap it and then you find that barely all that is left is the wallpapper. A support beam may look solid from the outside but proper inspection shows its interior is eaten away and it's ready to collapse.

A termite infestation strike hotels and produce dangerous results. Guide to causes and how to prevent their onslaught. You can tell when you've been visited by them. Termites usually shed their wings in groups and leave noticeable piles of these products of exfoliation. Another signal that termites are near is the presence of small pen-like mud tunnels running along the foundation of your hotel. Termites do not like the air and as a result, establish tunnels between the ground and your hotel. If you put an ice pick into a tunnel and it goes several inches into your hotel then it is likely that termite damage has been done and wood must be replaced. If the ice pick goes in less than an inch, the situation may be salvageable.

Salvageable only if you rid your land of termites, that is. Here is how to do it. The first and best option is the hire a professional. Fixing a bathroom faucet leak is a task that most hotelowners can and should attempt because the risk involved is low if you fail, but should the process of getting rid of termites fail the very foundation of your hotel is in danger. Professionals will tend to use the fumigation method which relies on the use of heavy-duty poisons.

If you must assume the exterminator role yourself here are some suggestions. You may use special insecticides. Drilling small holes into the diseased wood and pumping these chemicals in will kill the termites in several months. After the holes have been drilled you must fill them with caulk, however, to ensure that the termites are fully exposed to the death gas. Additionally, if you take boric acid dissolved in water and apply a layer to the wood termites will steer clear of your territory. Some people have found that using propane heat on the termites works as well. Professional guidance is recommended for this procedure, however. Freezing the bugs is safer and easier. Liquid nitrogen pumped into the wood will freeze the termites to death.

While these solutions may rid you of pests, the best solution is always prevention. Here are some ways of making sure your hotel is not a termite target. The most important thing to remember is a dry foundation is an inedible foundation; if you keep your wood dry you will not have a problem with termites. Avoid planting thirsty plants near the base of the hotel. Excess watering will attract termites if the wood retains the liquid. Avoid, if you can, building with woods termites find tasty, such as cedar and redwood. Digging a tiny tunnel (five inches deep) around your hotel and filling it with sand will block the passage to the wood as well.

There are products you can purchase at the hardware store that will protect your wood. Buy a wood preservative that contains pentachlorophenol and apply a few layers to the wood. Cover all the cracks and fissures to make sure it is completely insulated. Remember to remove any rotted wood you find so that the termites do not spread.

If you follow the above measures it is likely that your hotel will be safe. It is recommended however, if you have corroded wood that you seek professional help before you act. Sometimes rotten wood is an indicator of a dry rot. Dry rot is a microscopic fungus that, unlike its name suggests, is very wet. If the moisture of your wood is over twenty percent dry rot can appear. The air-borne fungus spreads quickly in wet conditions.

Feeding on the cellulose fibers of the wood, this fungus acts much like a termite. When the wood becomes very porous as a result of this hungry fungus it will absorb more and more water and will become weaker and weaker. At some point the weakness will translate into a crumbling foundation and a sloping, sinking, or crumbling hotel above. To prevent dry rot you can use the same methods as you would for keeping termites away. Remember, dry wood is happy termite-free, rot-free wood.

Cockroach Hotel Extermination

Cockroach hotel extermination can be accomplished through various methods. Discovering that cockroaches have invaded your hotel is a nightmare, to say the least. Roaches are often brought hotel in grocery bags, cardboard boxes, pet food bags, and in other items they can hide in. Cockroaches are often associated with dirty living conditions, but any hotel can become infested with cockroaches.

According to Mike Potter, cockroaches like locations that provide food, dampness, darkess, and warmth. He suggests making sure cardboard boxes, paper sacks, and pop bottles are not left around the hotel. He goes on to say, foods should be kept in sealed containers, and any spills or food particles should be cleaned up right away. Dirty dishes in the kitchen sink should be thoroughly rinsed or immediately washed after use. Kitchen garbage cans need to have sealed lids. Also, pet foods should not be left out. Cleanliness is important in preventing and getting rid of cockroaches, according to "Cockroach Elimination".

"Cockroach Elimination" recommends the use of boric acid and cockroach baits to help eliminate cockroaches. It says that baits are effective because cockroaches consume the bait and go back to their nests and die. Other roaches in the nest die from coming in direct contact with poisoned feces and sputum excreted by the dying cockroach. They are easy to use and are self-contained. The same article suggests placing baits in areas that cockroaches have been seen or are likely to go. The baits should be placed next to walls or corners and near crevices, since cockroaches are seldom out in the open. "Cockroach Elimination" says at least ten baits should be located in the kitchen and two in each bathroom. Two to four more baits should be used in other rooms where cockroaches have been sighted. Sprays should not be used in conjunction with baits since they may discourage cockroaches from going to the bait and ingesting it. Make sure extreme caution is used when placing cockroach bait or other insecticides where they can be reached by children and pets.

Boric acid powder is an odorless and highly effective product for controlling cockroaches, according to "Cockroach Elimination". However, it must be used correctly to be effective. The same article says it can be used simultaneously with cockroach baits. It goes on to say that boric acid does not deter cockroaches, so they will keep coming back to the treated area and eventually die.

Boric acid is also reported to be safe to use around children and pets. "Cockroach Elimination" says that boric acid should be used as a light dusting in areas frequented by cockroaches. Applying it too thickly will encourage them to go around it. Under appliances, sinks, and around plumbing are all common places to find cockroaches. It warns not to put boric acid in areas of food preparation or where the boric acid is visible.

If you give these methods time to work and do not achieve success, the infestation may be too advanced, and you will need to contact a professional exterminator.

Wood Boring Insects

Termites are the most damaging wood destroying insects and following closely in second place are wood boring beetles. Termites have straight torsos and antennae. The worker is without wings and grayish white in color. The solder has an exaggerated jaw. The reproductive termites are dark with wings forward and rear the same size. Other wood-boring insects include:

Carpenter Ants

The carpenter ant has a small middle section, shorter back wings, and bent antennae. A "stalk like stem" extends by the belly with one outgrowth. They burrow in decayed, moist, wood to make their nest. A good sign of infestation is left over grainy sawdust.

Caulking the exterior cracks is a good safeguard to help keep carpenter ants out of your hotel. Use weather-stripping in windows and doors. Work at preventing moisture problems in your hotel that attract these insects. Do not allow tree branches to brush against your hotel, and keep any fireplace wood a distance from your hotel. Replace decayed wood and keep gutters free from rotting wood, leaves, and debris.

POWDER-POST BEETLES

The true powderpost beetles are called, "Lyctid Powderpost Beetle," with over 30 species. Adults range up to ¼ inch long. Reddish brown to black in color they have slim bodies. They are limited to infestations in hardwood. You will notice a hole that is round in shape in the wood. The feeding beetle will leave a powdery dust behind, thus its name.

The immature form or larvae will actually damage the hardwood. Up to 50 eggs is laid by the female in crack on the ends of the boards. After hatching the larvae will tunnel to the lower surface of the wood and continue to grow into adults.

CARPENTER BEES

These look somewhat like bumblebees. Carpenter bees nest in burrows or tunnels in the outer surface of wood and can be found in wood trim, or facia and unfinished wood. After exterminating plug and refinish, the holes left behind with caulking, and refinish.

SUBTERRANEAN TERMITES

These termites are all throughout America and are the most common type, of termites. Their food is wood and the destruction and structural damage caused to a hotel can be extreme.

Termites nest under the ground, and pass through safety canals burrowed atop the ground to search for food above ground. They can invade the hotel by infesting wood that is untreated, or that touches the soil and joints that are not sealed correctly

Termites like moisture consequently keep your water sprinklers from splashing side of your hotel. Keep the soil from accumulating at the base of the foundation. Keep brush and foundation plantings away from air vents. Lumber should be pressure treated that is used to repair damaged wood next to the soil or concrete. A metal termite shield can be installed at the foundation while hotel is under construction. This will cause the termites to build on the outside of the foundation and can be easily inspected.

Control Measures

Most chemicals used for wood-boring insects are restricted and must be handled by licensed pest controllers Thes experts have access to a broader scope of insecticides and have the correct tools. The safer alternative would probably be to hire a professional for this sort of project.

Identifying Spiders Around the Hotel

Two most troublesome spiders are brown spiders and black widows both reclusive. Identifying which spider you have seen is important. If bitten what are the symptoms.

Most spiders cannot harm people, moreover are the stalkers of other pests, and are useful. Much of the populace have a distain for spiders, however their value ought to considered due to the fact that they help rid our hotels of unwanted insects. The spiders that could be harmful to people such as black widows, are usually hidden out of sight under objects in the hotel or in piles of wood out of doors. It is a usual rule that if a spider is out during the daylight hours, can be seen in your hotel, they are not the poisonous kind, and we need not be alarmed.

Many people refer to the spider as an insect, this is incorrect, and they are in fact arachnids. Spiders have two parts to their body and have eight legs, no wings, or antennae. Parts of the body are the sector near the head and the hind area referred to as their abdomen. Spiders eat mostly insects and other spiders but will occasionally be found on plants. Nearly all spiders have harmful venom, which is used to subdue their quarry, however the ones that have an effect on humans is due to an allergic reaction to the venom.

The jaws of most spiders are too small to pierce the skin of most grownups but tend to bite children more often. When a web is touched, deliberately or not, the vibration could cause a bite intuitively, the spider thinking it has caught an insect. A bite may cause little or no reaction to severe response, depending on such things as health and age of the person bitten. Some affects could be swelling, itching, redness, pain, and stiffness, but they are usually not too severe. However, if the bite causes extreme manifestations such as swelling and profound pain, call a physician!

There are times when an individual is not aware of having been bitten until they begin to notice pain and itching. Thes bites could be other arthropods, which include ticks, fleas, bedbugs, mosquitoes, flies, and such. In other words, spiders are not always to blame.

Pest control for Centipedes and Millipedes

Centipedes and millipedes may be annoying pests but are not dangerous. They can, however, invade your hotel when left untreated.

Centipedes and millipedes are seen commonly in yards and will occasionally enter hotels or buildings. Although both of these may be annoying or a bit frightening, neither of them is considered to be a real threat to humans. They do not cause harm to any inside or outside structures nor do they consume our food. In spite of this, however, excessive rain, drought, or lack of their food supply can bring about mass migrations that may lead to hotel invasions.

Centipedes (Chilopods) have flattened bodies with many segments and around one hundred legs. At least one pair of legs is attached to each body segment. They vary in length from one to six inches and can move rather quickly when bothered. Their eyesight is poor and are frequently seen at night. Centipedes are considered to be carnivorous as they are known to feed on spiders and other insects.

Even though centipedes may appear threatening, they are generally harmless to humans with exception to larger species which can inflict a painful and sometimes poisonous bite. Some people may experience an severe allergic reaction to its venom. For this reason, you should avoid handling any centipede. On average centipedes are associated with damp, dark places such as underneath leaves, rocks, bark, or mulch. On the other hand, the hotel centipede prefers the damp and high humidity areas found in basements, closets, bathrooms, and unexcavated regions under your hotel.

Millipedes (Diplopods) are more cylindrical with two pairs of legs attached to each body segment. They have thousands of legs but despite this, millipedes move slowly. Their bodies are adapted for burrowing instead of scurrying. Millipedes are also considered harmless, although they do coil up tightly if disturbed and secrete a foul-smelling fluid. These particular creatures often feed on damp and decaying wood, plant, and vegetable matter. As with centipedes, they are also most active at night and can be found under stones, flower pots, boards, or similar debris that is abundantly moist. Occasionally, millipedes will feed on living plant roots and developing fruits of cantaloupe or cucumbers. The affected plants will usually wilt and die. These pests are generally more troublesome in wooded or newly developed areas where decaying vegetation is more plentiful. They can, however, invade your hotel during wet seasons but usually die unless there is high moisture or a sufficient food source.

Centipedes and millipedes are not insects, but they are at times considered to be pests. They both live and breed in the same areas, but they each have different food sources. They typically become a nuisance when migrating and if left untreated they may infest your hotel and surroundings. Centipedes and millipedes are encouraged by wet conditions and controlling them involves both prevention and thorough treatment. Most common areas of invasion will occur alongside your hotel and in nearby mulch, compost or wood piles, and other moist locations. Knowing where to find these pests will make prevention and treatment easier.

Centipedes and millipedes can be prevented from gaining access into hotels and other structures by sealing any holes that might be around siding, windows, doors, or pipes. This can be done with caulking or weather stripping. They both require moist habitats and high humidity so it is important to keep your hotel and outside surroundings dry. Also keep trash, stones, old boards, leaves, grass clippings, and other debris away from your hotel. Removal of any thick mulch from your foundation and plants to allow drying will help reduce millipede problems. Dry conditions will make it difficult for them to feed and reproduce.

Watering lawns and gardens later in the day will also promote more drying out time. If there is a continuing presence of hotel centipedes in your hotel, this could actually signal an underlying insect problem. You may want to check your hotel for spiders, roaches, and other insects. Eliminating centipedes is less difficult when you take away their chief food source.

Since centipedes and millipedes are not considered insects, most insecticides do not work well with controlling migrations. However, using residual insecticide sprays along cracks, entry points, and baseboards may help discourage activity. You will want to spray thoroughly around foundations as well as the sides of structures. Be sure to get around the windows, across doorways, and other openings. Also, pay attention to plants, shrubs, and trees. Spray around the trunks and ground surrounding plants. The wet powder formulation generally provides the best soil control. Water thoroughly after treatment of mulches to allow insecticide to penetrate deeper into the soil. This is usually where any millipede nests may be found and will help keep them from developing. When using any insecticides, take the necessary precautions and always read carefully and follow label directions.

While both centipedes and millipedes may seem unpleasant, they are not dangerous. Although centipedes can sometimes inflict nasty bites, overall, they are quite beneficial. They are good predators of soil-dwelling pests, spiders, and other insects. Millipedes do not bite but do occasionally snack on various plant parts. However, they too provide a valuable service by breaking down organic matter. The good deeds of centipedes and millipedes far outweigh their indiscretions, and control is generally not necessary unless their population during migrations is unusually high.

Homemade Paper Wasp Trap

Paper wasps are beneficial insects, but they alarm people, and can become a nuisance. Trapping them in a homemade trap can reduce their numbers.

Paper wasps are a beneficial insect. Less aggressive than yellow jackets or hornets, they are useful in that they eat many harmful insects. They are called paper wasps because they construct umbrella shaped nests of a paper like material made of finely chewed wood fragments mixed with the wasps' salivary secretions. Paper wasps are social insects living in colonies, which can get quite large. They become a nuisance when they build their nests too near where people live.

While these large, slender, golden-brown wasps are reported to rarely sting, they are still unsettling to see skimming through the hotel, bumping the ceiling from time to time. They usually will fly to a window or an open door. If they get in a window that can't be opened, they can be gently crushed against the glass with a sturdy book, or you can do like my mother and cut their little waists with sewing scissors! But if that seems too savage, you might like to make a trap.

The best time to put a trap out is in the late winter or early spring. A paper wasp queen will hibernate through the winter, and come out with the first warm weather to start her new nest. If you catch a queen early, you might save yourself dealing with a thousand other worker wasps. Later in the year, you will probably need more than one trap, and by then it is unlikely that you will get rid of all the paper wasps.

A wasp trap is best located at least 20 feet from human activity areas and about 4 ft. above the ground. It should be moved as necessary to keep the temperature around 85 degrees F. Hang it in the shade on warmer days, and in the sun on cooler days.

An easy trap to make is from a plastic 2-liter pop bottle. Discard the lid. Cut the funnel shaped top off the bottle and save it. Fill the bottom with four inches of water and add a little dish soap. Add a little vinegar to discourage honeybees from visiting the trap. Attach bait (described below) to the threaded part of the funnel. Invert it into the bottom part of the bottle. Punch a few holes where the two pieces meet around the sides. Tie strings in these holes to make a hanger. Rub a little petroleum jelly around the opening so escaping wasps will lose their footing.

The basic idea behind the trap is to lure the wasp inside where they will wear themselves out trying to escape, and will fall into the water and drown. The soap in the water reduces surface tension, which in turn increases the likelihood of the insect suffocating.

In the late winter and early spring, wasps are attracted to protein bait, such as liverwurst, fish, or partially cooked hamburger, etc. Pet food is not a good choice, because the wasps will lose interest in it in a few days. In the summer, the wasps will be attracted to sweet foods, such as apple pieces or crushed grapes. But if the queens are trapped in the early spring, hopefully there won't be as much of a problem in the late summer.

Another wasp trap that can be easily constructed is to fill a 5-gallon bucket with water. Add some dish soap. Now suspend protein bait about an inch from the surface of the water. The wasps will try to carry off the heavy bait and will fall into the water and drown. If other animals' getting into the water is a problem, a cover can be made for the bucket out of wide mesh wire.

These traps need to be tended to frequently. In the trap made from a 2-liter bottle, the new wasps coming in can survive by resting on the wasps that have already drowned if there are two many of them still in the trap. In addition, if very many wasps find their way out, they might go back to the colony and cause a swarm. This happens when the colony believes it is being threatened, and the wasps become more aggressive and dangerous.

Crushing wasps' bodies should be avoided because they emit a chemical scent, which can act as an alarm to the others in their colony and cause agitation and swarming.

Hundreds of people die worldwide each year from wasp stings. As many as one in a thousand people have a serious allergy to stings. It is wise to avoid wasps and be careful not to excite them.

If it is necessary to knock down a nest, try to do it as early in the year as possible, when it is still small. It can be sprayed with a wasp freeze type of pesticide first. (Many sprays have an oily base and can damage surfaces on which they are sprayed.) Wear long sleeves and eye protection and don't stand directly under the nest. Do this at night, when the wasps are all hotel and sluggish from a hard day's work. Use a flashlight covered with red cellophane to decrease the stimulation to the wasps. Or hire a professional. If the queen survives, she is likely to go elsewhere to build her next nest.

In the event of a sting, carefully wash the sting site with cool water. Vinegar is reported to ease the pain of a sting. Then apply antihistamine cream. If antihistamine cream is unavailable, use a little meat tenderizer or baking soda mixed with a little water. This will draw the poison out and help remove the stinger. Be aware that a wasp can sting more than once. In fact, a dead wasp on the ground can inject its stinger into a nearby bare foot! If the patient is known to be allergic to stings, or if they begin to feel sleepy, get medical help immediately.

Hornets and yellow jackets make a paper-like nest, too, which is usually shaped like an upside-down teardrop and found in trees. Yellow jackets sometimes make their nests in old rodent burrows in the ground. Both of these wasp species are more aggressive and dangerous than paper wasps, and should be left to the professional for removal.

Mud daubers are the least aggressive of the wasps. They usually make their earthen hotels inside barns or other structures away from human activity. They do not live in large colonies and are usually not a problem. In addition, they eat many other harmful insects.

When possible, it is good to leave wasps alone, since they provide a valuable service. When they get too close to the hotel, though, they cause trouble. A thoughtfully placed trap can help remove them.

Controlling and Killing Rats and Mice

Sometimes, no matter how clean your hotel is mice or rats can move in with you. They are dirty and germ carrying and they are extremely damaging to your hotel and its contents. They are annoying and can be noisy too. You can be certain you have a mouse or rat problem if you see the small black droppings along walls and under counters and in closets. Or if you see the rodent itself— you know you have a problem. They will chew up your clothes and anything else that they can get to use to make a nest. Here is what you can do to rid this nuisance.

Mice can fit through the tiniest of holes. You should check for cracks or holes leading outside or under your hotel. Mice usually enter in pipes leading into the hotel through floors and will enter through any other holes as well. You should check under all kitchen and bathroom cabinets for holes. Also check around gas lines and other lines that run into your hotel. If you find any holes you can fill them with steel wool, this may deter the mice until you can take more permanent precautions. Caulking is excellent to use to close up small holes. Check your cabinets frequently to assure that no pests have attempted to chew through; though this is quite unlikely.

If your hotel is already infested with mice there are plenty of options to rid your hotel of these pests. You can use the standard spring back mouse traps to kill mice. These traps can be messy, so they may not be for everyone. They are also dangerous if you have pets or children. The spring traps can injure them. Sticky glue traps are a great option. They are also a bit more humane. The mouse will be attracted by the smell of the trap and when he gets on the trap—he is stuck. You can let the mouse loose if you choose. You should also keep glue traps out of reach from pets and children. Remember to place traps along baseboards right up against the walls, as this is where mice travel.

Mice and rats are effectively controlled with poisons. The only problem with poison is that you often do not find the mouse until he is dead and producing that retched odor. Pets can also be harmed if they ingest a poisoned animal. Of course you should not let your pets or children anywhere near the poison.

Rats, on the other hand are not as common as mice when it comes to infestation. Rats will live anywhere and will eat anything. This means that your hotel is not immune to rats. They are mostly controlled by poisoning. You should take care to guard against a rat infestation. Follow the same steps as in preventing mice. Fill all holes under cabinetry. Make sure all openings to the crawl space under your hotel are all covered with no openings. Do not keep anything stacked against your hotel; such as a wood pile. Rats can hide in small spaces and can set up a nest anywhere. Never keep garbage around your hotel. Use sealed, lidded trash cans, since trash can and will attract rats and mice. A dog or cat is also a good consideration. Cats are more known for catching mice, but dogs will get in on the action as well.

Rats and mice are disgusting little animals when they enter your hotel uninvited. Having one or the other as a pet can be a different scenario! When they infest your hotel, they can infect it as well by carrying germs and diseases. Rats are particularly infamous for plagues and rabies. Take caution when trying to exterminate rats on your own. With rats, you should seek out a professional.

You should also seek a pro with an out of control mouse infestation. Exterminators can come in and help you find the points of entry but you will be responsible for fixing this—they just place the poison. Pest control companies will often offer you a contract for them to exterminate and prevent re-infestations on a monthly basis. The good thing about using a professional is that most of the time their work is guaranteed. When you have a problem like rats or mice—a guarantee is a great asset.

Bibliography

Cichy, Ronald F., "Managing Service in Food and Beverage Operations", Lansing: Educational Institute of the American Hotel and Motel Association, 1998.

__________., "Quality Sanitation Management", East Lansing: Educational Institute of the American Hotel & Motel Association, 1994.

Clark, Mona, *Interpersonal Skills for Hospitality Managers*, London: Chapman Hill, 1995.

McDonnell, Jane, *Step By Step Art of Table Decorating*, New York: Crescent Books, 1994.

McSwane, David Zachary, *Essentials of Food Safety and Sanitation*, Upper Saddle River: Prentice Hall, 2000.

Mills, Irving J., *Tabletop Presentations: A Guide for the Foodservice Professional*, New York: Van Nostrand Reinhold, 1989.

Nam, Inja, *Art of Garnishing*, New York: Van Nostrand Reinhold, 1993.

Ninemeier, Jack D., "Management of Food and Beverage Operations", East Lansing: Educational Institute of the American Hotel and Motel Association, 1995.

__________., "Planning and Control for Food and Beverage Operations", Orlando: Educational Institute, 1998.

Notarius, Barbara, *Open Your Own Bed & Breakfast*. New York: John Wiley & Sons, Inc., 1996.

Nykiel, Ronald A., "Marketing in the Hospitality Industry", East Lansing: Educational Institute of the American Hotel and Motel Association, 1997.

Peterson, James, *Sauces: Classical and Contemporary Sauce Making*, New York: Van Nostrand Reinhold, 1998.

Rande, Wallace L., *Introduction to Professional Foodservice*, New York: Wiley, 1996.

Reed, Lewis, "Specs: The Comprehensive Foodservice Purchasing and Specification Manual", Van Nostrand Reinhold, 1993.

Riley, Michael, "Managing People: A Guide for Managers in the Hotel and Catering Industry", Oxford: Butterworth Heinemann, 1995.

Index